Ultrasound Services in an Early Pregnancy and Acute Gynaecological Unit
Book 1

© Oluwakemi O. Ola – Ojo
2018

Dedication

This book is dedicated to:
You,
Our past and present students.
Thank you all for allowing my colleagues and me to share with you from our
wealth of knowledge and experience
and
To all my colleagues from the multidisciplinary team,
it has been a blessing working with you all. Thanks.

Manasseh

"For God has made me forget all my trouble and hardship"
Genesis 41:51. - Amplified Bible Version

First published 2018
ISBN: 978-1-908015-07-5
British Library Cataloguing in Publication Data
A catalogue record for this book is available from the British Library

Library of Congress Cataloguing in Publication Data

Design: Redsorel Designs

Acknowledgements

I would like to express my profound thanks to the following organisations: Royal Free Hospital NHS Trust London –my employer. Ectopic Trust for allowing me to use their illustration of ectopic pregnancy locations. GE Healthcare for allowing me to use the images of their ultrasound probes and sterilisation process. I am grateful to HealthNetConnections and GE Healthcare for providing the access to the obstetrics charts reference data & respective authors; which are used within their Viewpoint ultrasound reporting software.

A million thanks to Dr Peter Wylie, Consultant Radiologist for allowing me to use the MRI images and for reviewing book 2 of the series; Mr Khaled Zaedi, Consultant Obstetrician & Gynaecologist for reviewing book 1 of the series; Dr Phyllis Serbang, then Radiology Registrar for reviewing both books, providing wise counsel and encouragement. To my colleagues who shared their interesting cases with me, I am most grateful.

To two of our 'then' newly qualified sonographers whose quest for excellence in EPAGU ultrasound led to the writing of these books, I am grateful for your trust, commitment to learning and good practice.

Thank you to all the multidisciplinary team members involved in setting up and running the EPAGU services, for their dedication and commitment especially those of the Doctors, Nurses, Administrative and House Keeping staff, Laboratory staff and FMU staff.

To all the students, colleagues and your good self who have made writing this book worthwhile. I am very grateful.

Finally and not in the least, to my family and friends – your understanding, prayers and support have been remarkable. Thank you all.

Contents

Chapter 3   77

Chapter 4   169

Book Reviews

"This is a great effort and dedication on illustration of the ultrasound images and explanation of findings. The author has taken time in explaining different scenarios with the aid of ultrasound images. The case reviews are interesting and logically approached."

Mr. Khaled Zaedi
Consultant Obstetrician & Gynaecologist
EPAGU Consultant lead, Royal Free London NHS Trust

"All ultrasound trainees both medical and non-medical should get their hands on this book, which provides a comprehensive guide to gynaecology/obstetrics ultrasound and can be used as a first reader for ultrasound trainees and referred to throughout the course of training."

Phyllis Nsiah- Sarbeng
Then Radiology Registrar, Royal Free London NHS Trust

Abbreviations

3-D	–	3-dimensional
4-D	–	4-dimensional
AC	–	Abdominal circumference
A&E	–	Accident & Emergency
AF	–	Amniotic fluid
AFI	-	Amniotic fluid index
AGEPU	–	Acute gynaecological and early pregnancy unit
AGU	–	Acute gynaecological unit
AM	–	Amniotic membrane
ANC	–	Antenatal clinic
a/40 a =		gestational age/40. 40 = average length of a normal pregnancy
AP	–	Anteroposterior
b+c/40	–	b=number of weeks + c = days.
BMUS	–	British Medical Ultrasound Society
BPD	–	Biparietal diameter
bpm	–	beats per minute
CD	–	Compact disk
CH	–	Clinical history
CI	–	Cord insertion
CLC	–	Corpus luteal cyst
COR	–	College of Radiographers
CP	–	Choroid plexus
CRL	–	Crown-rump length
c/s	–	Caesarean section
CVS	–	Chorionic villus sampling
c/52	–	c = number of weeks. 52 = weeks per year
DA	–	Diamniotic
DAU	–	Day assessment unit
DC	–	Dichorionic
DCDA	–	Dichorionic diamniotic
EDD	–	Expected date of delivery
EHR	–	Embryonic heart rate
EMB	–	Embryonic heart beat

EMP – Embryonic pole
EP – Ectopic pregnancy
EPAGU – Early pregnancy and acute gynaecology unit
EPU – Early pregnancy unit
FET – Frozen embryo transfer
FH – Fetal head
FHB – Fetal heart beats
FL – Femur length
FMU – Fetal medicine unit
FP – Fetal pole
GA – Gestational age
GH – Gut herniation
GIFT – Gamete intrafallopian transfer
GIT – Gastrointestinal tract
GP – General practitioner
GS – Gestational sac
GSD – Gestational sac diameter
GSV – Gestational sac volume
HC – Head circumference
HCG – Human chorionic gonadotropin
ICSI – Intracytoplasmic sperm injection
IPAD – Touch screen tablet PC made by Apple
IUCD – Intrauterine contraceptive device
IUD – Intrauterine death
IUGS – Intra uterine gestational sac
IUI – Intrauterine insemination
IUP – Intrauterine pregnancy
IVF – In vitro fertilisaton
KUB – Kidneys, ureters and bladder
LIF - Left illiac fossa
LLB – Lower limb bud
LMP – Last menstrual period
LS – Longitudinal section
LT – Left
LUQ - Left upper quadrant

MA   –   Missed abortion/miscarriage
MC   –   Monochorionic
MCDA – Monochorionic diamniotic
MCMA – Monochorionic monoamniotic
M mode – Motion mode
MTD -   Multi Disciplinary meeting
MTOP -   Medical termination of pregnancy
NHS   –   National Health Service
NICE –   National Institute for Health and Care Excellence
NT   –   Nuchal translucency
OHSS –   Ovarian hyperstimulation syndrome
PACS –   Picture archiving computer system
PCO -   Polycystic ovary
PCOS –   Polycystic ovary syndrome
PID   –   Pelvic inflammatory disease
PM   –   Postmenopausal
PMH –   Past medical history
POD –   Pouch of Douglas
PROM – Premature rupture of the membranes
PUL   –   Pregnancy of unknown location
PV   –   Per vagina
RCOG – Royal College of Obstetricians and Gynaecologists
RIF   -   Right illiac fossa
RPOC – Retained products of conception
RSI   –   Repetitve strain injury
RUQ -   Right upper quadrant
SROM – Spontaneous rupture of the membrane
STOP -   Surgical termination of pregnancy
RT   –   Right
R/V   –   Retroverted
SUZI –   Subzonal insemination
TA   –   Trans-abdominal
TS   –   Transverse section
TOP -   Termination of pregnancy
TTTS – Twin-to-twin transfusion syndrome

TV   –   Trans-vaginal
UKAS –   United Kingdom Association of Sonographers
ULB   –   Upper limb bud
VD   –   Vitelline duct
WC   –   Water closet
YS   –   Yolk sac
<   –   Less than
>   –   Greater than
=   –   Equal to

Introduction

It is unrealistic to present in this book all the possible normal and abnormal findings seen in an early pregnancy and acute gynaecology unit (EPAGU), or acute gynaecological and early pregnancy unit (AGEPU), but these have been provided as examples. Sometimes it is not possible to obtain standard ultrasound views due to many factors, but those presented in this book are the best obtainable views. Where the outcome is known in each of the cases presented, it will be mentioned.

For ease of writing and clarifications in this book, the ultrasonographer/ sonographer will be referred to as he/him, whilst the patient will be referred to as she/her.

Many protocols govern ultrasound examination practices from organisations such as NICE, BMUS, RCOG, COR, UKAS, and hospitals including that of chaperoning etc. The sonographer is encouraged to get familiar with his departmental protocols. The charts used may not be the same for all departments. Please refer to your own departmental charts.

Chapter 1

Setting up ultrasound services in EPAGU

This chapter will address the following:

Definitions

An ultrasound unit in EPAGU

How to go about setting up the ultrasound service in EPAGU

Reception and Patients waiting area

Ultrasound room

Patient's ensuite toilet

Counselling room

Recording of ultrasound examinations

Unit policies

Unit protocols

Patients information leaflets

Sources of patients

Methods of scanning

Sale of ultrasound pictures

Reporting package

Safety considerations

Quality issues

Benefits of having a dedicated ultrasound service in EPAGU

After the new set - up- what next?

Definitions:

AGU   –   Acute gynaecological unit

EPU   –   Early pregnancy unit. In some hospitals, the unit doubles up as AGU/ EPU and is therefore referred to as either:

EPAGU –   Early pregnancy and acute gynaecological unit

or as

AGEPU –   Acute gynaecological and early pregnancy unit

For ease of writing and reading, I will be using EPAGU from now on.

An ultrasound unit in EPAGU

Formerly, it was not unusual for the ultrasound room and ultrasound equipment to be allocated to any space or corridor in the X-ray/ANC departments of a hospital with little consideration for staff and service users. Over the years, healthcare providers have listened to their clients and things have and are still changing. Government guidelines from NICE and professional bodies such as RCOG and COR mean that many hospitals have or are in the process of organising a dedicated EPAGU, and ultrasound service is an essential part of any dedicated EPAGU.

The EPAGU is usually a unit of its own, separate from FMU, ANC and the radiology ultrasound department. It is separate from the unit that provides the NT screening programme. It is not in the gynaecology clinic or ward, or in the community gynaecology unit, nor is it in the A&E department. It should, however, be accessible by all these clinics and wards and by GPs. It is also separate from the Day Assessment Unit (DAU) that deals with problems seen in advanced pregnancy (after 20 weeks' gestation, 20/40 GA).

Ultrasound is the first imaging modality used in the biological female pelvic assessment, for many gynaecological and obstetric conditions. This is because of the following features: it is non-invasive, never contraindicated, does not use ionising radiation, never needs to observe the '10-day rule' (confine radiological examination of pelvis or lower abdomen to 10 days after menstruation) and can be done any time in the woman's cycle. Ultrasound is easily available in hospitals across the United Kingdom and can be used to monitor many obstetric and gynaecological events and situations that can confront patients. It must, however, be stressed that the use and interpretation of ultrasound examinations is operator dependent.

How to go about setting up the ultrasound service in EPAGU

Once the need has been identified and the provisions and commitment for ultrasound facilities have been recognised, the parties proposing the set-up will need to have many multilevel meetings including the following members of the hospital staff: consultant obstetricians and gynaecologists, gynaecology ward and clinic matron, ultrasound manager, clinical lead for ultrasound, the hospital works department, finance department, architects and building engineers, the hospital management team, and GP fundholders. Good communication is essential throughout the process if the set-up is to be successful.

The ultrasound manager or his representative will need to make time for attending the various planning meetings and site meetings. Whatever is agreed at such meetings needs to be documented and followed up.

It is important to plan to provide services and facilities that will meet the immediate and future needs and expectations of the service user and providers. Good communication is essential throughout the process if the set-up is to be successful.

Design of the ultrasound suite

Apart from the main EPAGU reception, a separate reception may not be needed for ultrasound. The reception and patients' waiting area can be in the same area/space jointly shared with the EPAGU staff and manned by the same administrative staff. The patient waiting or reception area should be spacious, well lit, have facilities for drinking water such as water filtering machines and disposable cups. Children, who might have to come with their mothers, should have a dedicated furnished play area. There should be a toilet and baby changing facilities in or around the reception area.

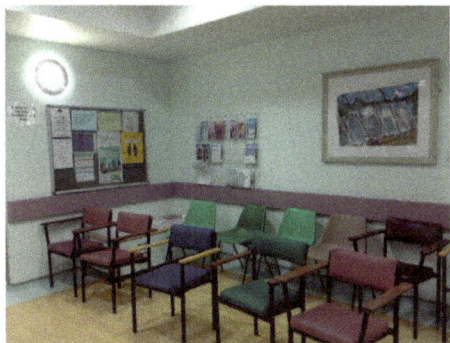

1a

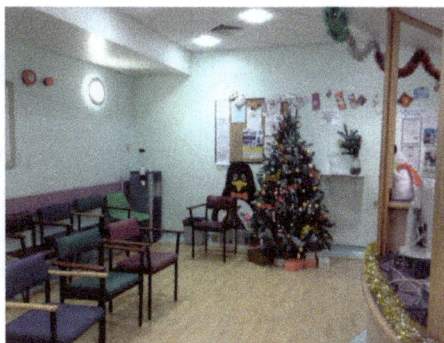

1b

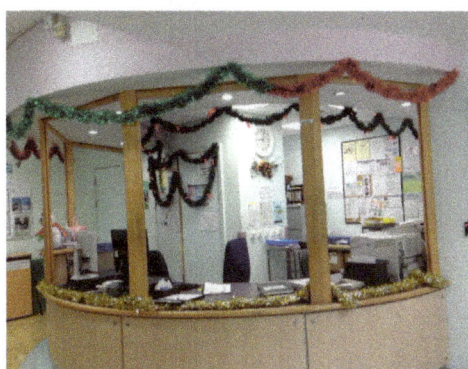

1c

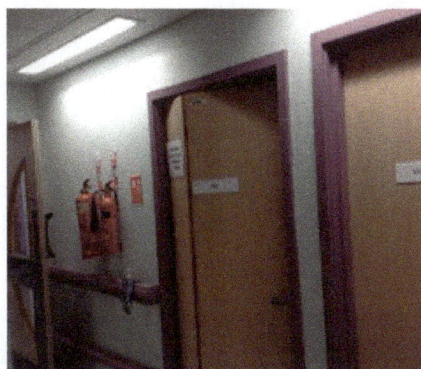

1d

An example of EPAGU reception, patient's waiting area and toilets from various angles

Ultrasound room

The design of the ultrasound room(s) within the EPAGU will be influenced by the size of the available space. However, there are guidelines that specify acceptable room dimensions. The number of ultrasound rooms needed will be determined by the current and anticipated patient workload. It is estimated that an ultrasound room can cope with approximately 5000 mixed routine examinations per year. Blackout and a dimmable lighting system will be required in the room together with an examination light.

Whatever the design that is chosen, the ultrasound room entrance should be large enough for patients who might have to come on a normal or bariatric hospital bed, stretcher or wheelchair including bariatric bed or bariatric wheelchair. There should be enough space in the ultrasound room to safely manoeuvre and accommodate a normal or bariatric hospital bed, stretcher or wheelchair. At least of the ultrasound rooms, should have enough space for a bariatic bed or wheelchair.

In a consultant-led unit, it is advisable to have at least two ultrasound rooms – one of the ultrasound rooms for the clinician to use as a consulting and ultrasound room and the other room for the ultrasonographer.

An example of an ultrasound room from various angles

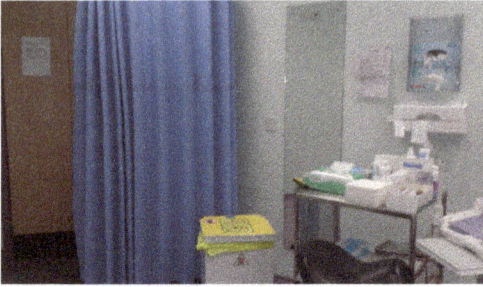 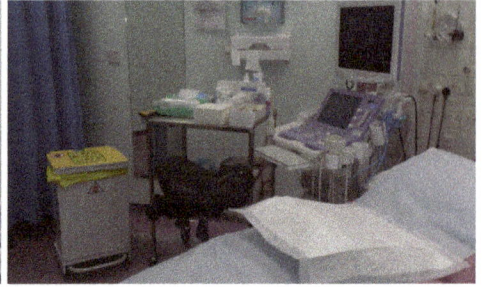

1e   *Scanning set up and sundries*   **1f**

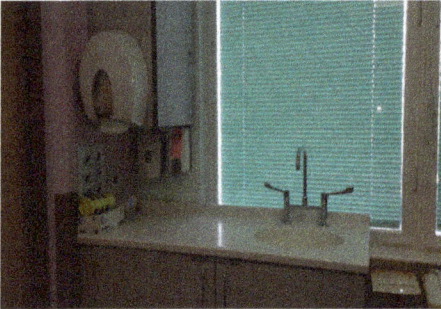 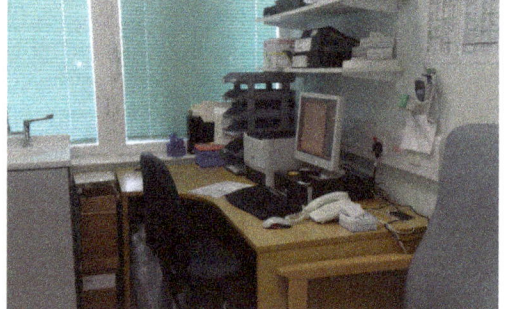

1g   *Wash hand sink*   **1h** *Sonographer's reporting area*

Example of another ultrasound room but with different arrangements

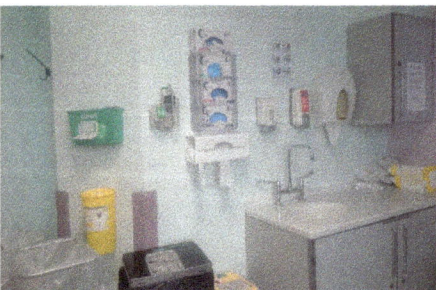 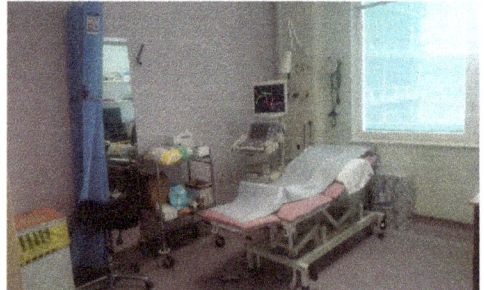

1i   **1j**

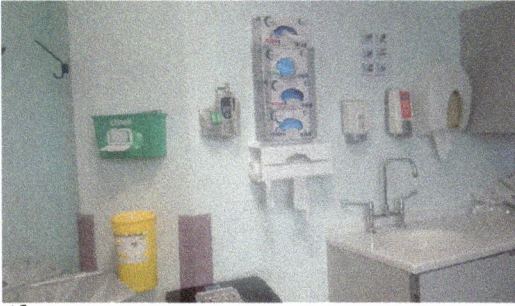 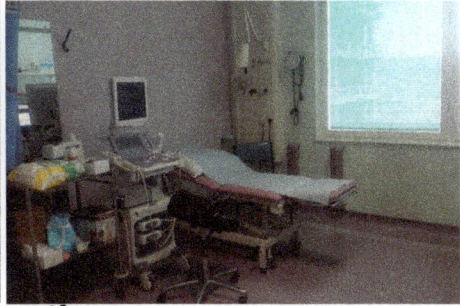

1k   1l

There is no good or bad way, it will depend on the sonographers' preferences

Equipment and accessories for the ultrasound room

The ultrasound manager and his team will need to produce a list of the equipment and accessories that will be needed. These may include the following in no particular order:

- Pillows
- A telephone
- TV probe covers
- Dimmable lighting
- Ultrasound equipment
- Patients' gowns or sheets.
- Pillow slips and couch cover
- Ultrasound gel bottles (filled)
- Emergency call button or switch
- A computer with ultrasound reporting package
- Disposable blue rolls or reusable sheets for the couch
- A printer and facilities for printing the ultrasound reports
- One or two chairs for patients' husband or partner or relative
- Ultrasound gel bottle warmer for TA scan especially in winter
- Scanning couch with facilities for varying the height and possible head tilt
- Scanning pad or stirrups or an extra chair for patients' feet to rest upon
- Facilities for storing copies of the ultrasound images and reports, e.g. paper, thermal paper, CDs
- Facilities for linking the ultrasound equipment with PACS or hospital data or picture base
- Separate TV screen for the patient and relatives to watch the examination

- A desk for the computer or facilities for writing ultrasound reports
- A chair for the ultrasonographer to use whilst working on the computer. This chair should be on wheels, adjustable in height and comfortable to sit on thus keeping the spine straight
- A sonographer's scanning stool which has facilities for varying its height and keeping the sonographer's spine straight and improving posture, e.g. a saddle seat
- Facilities for hard copies for patients, e.g. thermal/polaroid printer and relevant print paper
- Orange-yellow lined bins
- Red bags for blood-soiled linen
- Paper towels, sheets and incontinent pads
- Facilities for cleaning blood and body fluids
- Facilities for cleaning the ultrasound probes especially the TV probe
- Rubber gloves (small, medium, large) – be aware of sensitivity to latex both for ultrasonographers and patients
- Wash hand basin, soap, disposable hand papers (towels) and cream dispensers
- Facilities for having all the scanning sundries within easy reach, e.g. a nearby trolley

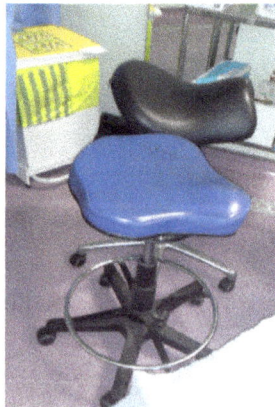

1m
Examples of sonographer's scanning stools

Which ultrasound equipment?

The choice and selection ultrasound equipment used will be determined by many factors, including, transportable ultrasound equipment from another arm of the hospital to a new set-up, or the purchasingor hiring of new equipment. When the new equipment is to be purchased or hired, the selection will be influenced by the available funds; if needs be, additional staff training; the user-friendliness of the equipment; the quality or resolution of the images on screen and hard copy; the ability to upgrade it in the future, e.g. to 3-D or 4-D; its compatibility with the existing hospital reporting package; the ease of moving the ultrasound equipment/ machine if and when the need arises; the ability to link the examination to PACS, or upgrade to that in the future.

Some hospitals use one or more ultrasound equipment manufacturers, whilst others are happy to buy or hire from many manufacturers. This may be through a hospital's rolling capital equipment replacement programme so that, at all times, modern ultrasound equipment is provided for all obstetric and gynaecological examinations. Both have their advantages and disadvantages. What is important is that the best equipment is purchased or hired according to requirements and possible future expansion.

There are other essentials that must be addressed when choosing ultrasound equipment or machine. These include the following:
- It has cine-loop facilities
- It has high or good image resolution
- It has multi frequency TA and TV probes
- It has a good and reliable breakdown/service agreement
- It has Doppler facilities – M mode, Colour/Power Doppler
- The keyboard, annotation, measurement facilities are very much user-friendly
- It has the relevant obstetric charts as used in the hospital or can have the hospital charts loaded onto it
- It has been used for less than 5 years unless it has been upgraded to make it compatible with expectations in relation to the quality of the images produced

- It is 3-D or 4-D compatible or can be upgraded to these scanning planes. This might require some extra training for the ultrasonographers in the unit
- 3-D/4-D are gradually finding their way into gynaecology scans. Where the ultrasonographer is familiar with its use and image interpretation, it is helpful especially in demonstrating and diagnosing uterine abnormalities and ectopic pregnancies

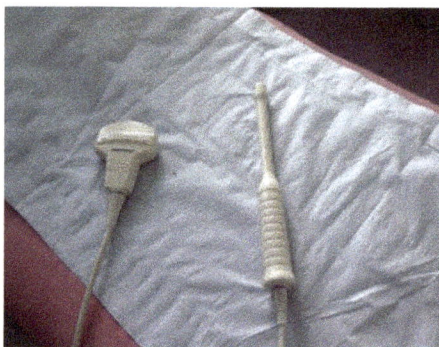 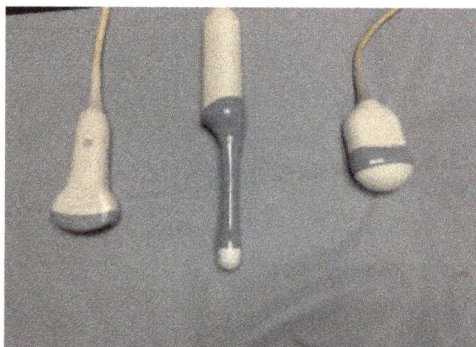

1n   *Examples of TA and TV probes*   *1o*

En Suite Toilet

It is essential to have a patient's toilet adjacent/attached to each ultrasound room (en-suite) so that less time is wasted in patients changing or using the toilet before or during the ultrasound examination. The toilet can serve as the changing room so the patient can have her privacy, whilst changing before or after a TV scan. This toilet is different to the one in the patients' waiting room (area).

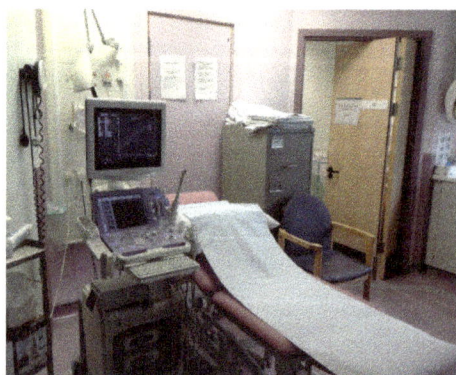 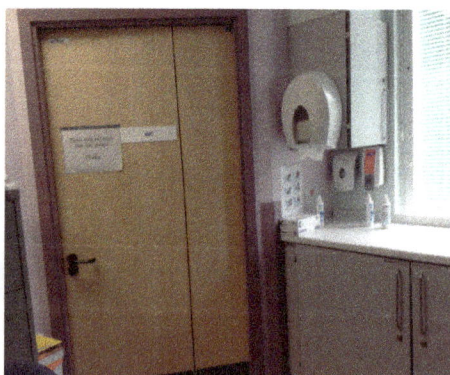

1p   *1q*

An example of an Ultrasound room and door leading to en-suite toilet

Equipment and accessories for the toilet -not in any particular order

- Wash hand basin
- Sanitary towels bin
- Standard or disabled WC
- Toilet rolls and holders
- Orange-yellow-lined bins
- Hand paper towels, soap, cream and their dispensers
- Sanitary accessories such as disposable knickers and pads
- Specimen bottles as the nurse or doctor may need urine samples
- White dirty linen laundry bag for used but unstained or uncontaminated linen
- Red dirty linen laundry bags for blood and body fluid-soiled or contaminated linen

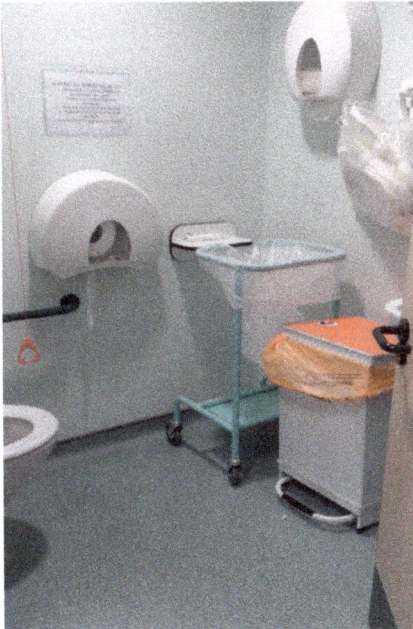

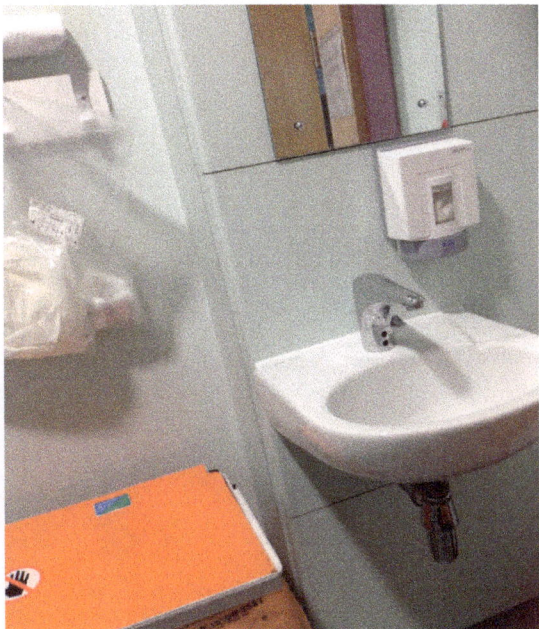

1r   1s

An example of an en-suite toilet

Counselling room

It is essential that there should be a dedicated counselling room, where couples given 'bad obstetric news' following their scan can have their privacy and space, whilst waiting for the midwife and/or doctor to see them. In addition, this room should be away from the waiting room. Ideally this room should be located adjacent to the ultrasound room so that couples who need their privacy post-ultrasound examination can do so without having to walk through the reception or busy patient areas.

What equipment and accessories will be needed in the counselling room?

Rather than having to sit amongst others in the waiting area, a patient who has been given bad news may often want to be by herself to cry, grieve, think of questions to ask and perhaps call her next of kin if there is no one else with her at the time of the scan. She may be very upset and shocked. A comfortable, uncluttered counselling room is useful at a time like this. This room should be located within the unit. It should be of adequate size with at least a table (where the clinician can write) and have chairs for the clinician, midwife, patient and her husband or partner. There should be some tissues, a rack of information leaflets and perhaps a telephone.

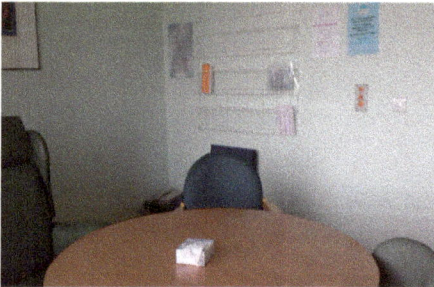

1t

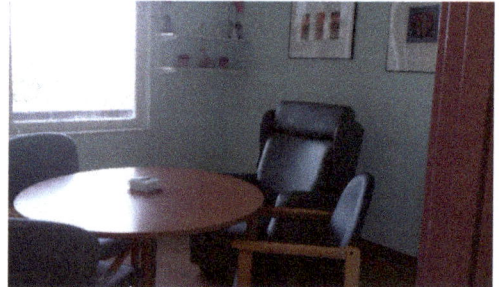

1u

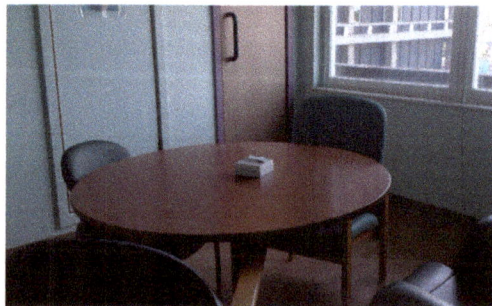

1v

An example of a counselling room from various angles

Recording of ultrasound examinations

Patients who want a photo of their baby are asked to give a token towards this service provided. Prices vary between different hospitals. In some hospitals there is a token/stamp machine where the patient puts the money and it gives them the token for the picture. In most NHS hospitals recording on videotapes or on a phone or iPad is not allowed. The College of Radiographers (COR), to which many sonographers belong, does not approve of such recordings. Ultrasound departments should have a protocol on what is acceptable, that is, a large notice clarifying the hospital's policy regarding filming or non-filming of ultrasound examinations.

Others

The dirty linen room, staff room can be shared by the ultrasonographers and the other members of the EPAGU team.

What else will be needed in the unit?

Unit policies

These are in line with hospital and current professional guidelines. Policies on the type of acceptable requests and from whom: Who is qualified to scan in the unit; TV scanning; confirmation of intrauterine death – by one or two sonographers; same sex chaperoning; reporting, giving information on findings; how many people can stay for a gynaecology or obstetric scan; what is expected in each scan; when and who to refer to if and when needed; video recording; how long to keep scan records for; routine equipment maintenance and fault reporting; thermal prints for patients and the cost per picture to the patient. In most NHS hospitals recording on videotapes or on the phone or iPads is not allowed. The COR does not approve of such recordings. There should be a large display notice in the patients' waiting area and in the ultrasound room clarifying the hospital's policy regarding filming or non-filming of ultrasound examinations.

Unit protocols

Protocols on what is acceptable in the ultrasound department should be in operation. Such protocols should outline guidelines in relation to sterilisation and disinfection of equipment, instruments and materials, especially the probes, what is expected in each obstetric or gynaecology ultrasound report. All the relevant protocols for ultrasound scanning should be in a file that is available in the ultrasound room for new or agency sonographers and for quick referencing if and when it is needed as well sonographer orientation booklet. Policies and protocols that are being used will enhance the service provided across the board and promote good team spirit.

There is need to have sonographer's orientation leaflet.

Patient information leaflets

It is also useful to have patient information leaflets on what to expect when having an ultrasound scan as well as other leaflets for such medical conditions as:

- Miscarriage
- Ovarian cysts
- Molar pregnancy
- Ectopic pregnancy
- Missed abortion or miscarriage
- Pregnancy of Unknown Location (PUL)

When the above leaflets are being designed, there should be input from the consultant obstetricians, gynaecologists, the ward and clinic matrons, who are likely to be in contact with patients. Ultrasound manager should also be involved as should some of the patients who have previously experienced the above conditions, but subsequently had a normal pregnancy and delivery. Such patients can provide an insightful view of their experiences and identify questions which they would have wanted to be answered or information that might have been helpful to them at the time they had complications.

Each leaflet should have the following information

- Title of the information leaflet
- Without using medical jargon, what the condition means
- Incidence rates nationally or locally if known. Otherwise the patient may feel abnormal
- Possible causes of the condition, if known
- Possible available ways for managing the condition in your hospital
- Effects on a future pregnancy if any

- Useful hospital or local contact telephone numbers
- Role of ultrasound in the management of any future pregnancy
- Available local and national support telephone numbers or organisations and their websites
- Relevant and useful websites

Each patient information leaflet should be written in relation to the literacy level of the general population being served. For hospitals with a large multicultural population, such leaflets may need to be made available in the various major languages of the population being served and printed on an ad hoc basis for the individual patient.

Information leaflets can provide uniform advice to all patients with the same clinical condition in that hospital. Patients and their families can refer to this information later, especially when the husband or partner is not available or present at the time of the ultrasound examination, or where the patient needs to clarify any information about her ultrasound findings. Information leaflets thus provide useful contact details for a patient and her family. In addition, the leaflets help to eliminate any errors of not providing enough information to the patient at the time of the scan by any team member, therefore promoting a good team spirit in a multidisciplinary team.

The advantage of having a hospital patient information leaflet as opposed to those generated by the various charities is that the hospital-generated information leaflets will provide more answers to the immediate questions of the couple about who to contact, and further possibilities that can be pursued in that particular hospital.

Sources of patients

Patients in need of an early pregnancy ultrasound scan or an acute gynaecological scan may be referred to the unit up to 18/40 by the following medical personnel or their relevant departments:

- Local GPs
- Community midwives
- Hospital consultants

- Clinical manager ANC
- Hospital A&E department
- Patients with a bad obstetric history can self-refer

* Referral to EPAGU is usually by phone, fax or mail.

Methods of scanning

This will depend on why we are scanning. Patients needing an emergency gynaecology ultrasound and where they are not nil by mouth (i.e. can eat and drink), should ideally attend the examination with a full bladder so that a trans-abdominal scan is performed first before embarking on the trans-vaginal scan. With the trans-abdominal scan, we can obtain a 'helicopter' view of the pelvis, which is particularly useful in assessing huge fibroids, pelvic cyst(s) and mass (es). There is also a lot of space for the ultrasonographer to manoeuvre the trans-abdominal probe. However, where the patient is in a condition of nil by mouth or is vomiting or in an emergency when there is no time for having a full bladder, the trans-abdominal scan may have to be suspended. Scanning a patient using the TA approach allows the sonographer a wider range or room for manoeuvre, unlike a TV scan.

Trans-vaginal ultrasound scans provide 'close-up views' of the pelvic organs, which can be helpful, where the concern is about fine details. This form of scan does not need a full urinary bladder. In fact, it is ideal for the patient who is vomiting, cannot keep fluids down, is nil by mouth, cannot have a full bladder, or in a dire emergency when there is urgent need to diagnose what is wrong with the patient or clarify the findings of a trans-abdominal scan. However, there may be limitations or difficulties of moving the trans-vaginal probe sufficiently to obtain all the views needed.

In many early pregnancy units the protocol is to have the patient produce a urine sample before the ultrasound scan is done, thus making a trans-vaginal scan the first option or choice. With this method, a normal early pregnancy can be visualised approximately one week earlier than when a trans-abdominal scan is used.

Preparing for a trans-abdominal pelvic scan

The patient lies down in the supine position on the examination couch. The pelvic area is exposed from the bikini line to the umbilicus. A paper towel is tucked into the patient's knickers. Some warm gel is applied to the abdomen. The urinary bladder should be identified in the longitudinal section and that serves as a good landmark for the pelvic organs to be correctly identified and assessed. The whole length and width of each organ should be examined and documented as well as the echo texture or pattern of each structure. Any abnormality or variant should be documented in both the images obtained and in the written report.

Preparing for a trans-vaginal pelvic scan

Prior to this examination, the patient is informed what the examination will entail. A verbal or written informed consent is obtained as stipulated by the unit's protocol and sensitivity to latex is confirmed. Whilst all pregnant patients are suitable for a TV scan if needed, not all patients for emergency gynaecology ultrasound are and this must be checked and must not be assumed. The intimate nature of the trans-vaginal scan, if not practised in a sensitive and respectful manner, may lead to misinterpretation. Sonographers should be sensitive to the needs of their patients and be aware of the potential impact of their actions.

Privacy and the presence of a chaperone should be provided and documented, in line with the hospital policy. The patient is allowed to empty her urinary bladder just prior to the scan. She is told to undress only from the waist down, a small basket or disposable bag should be provided for her to put her clothes in. She should be offered a patient gown to change into with the opening of the gown at the back or a sheet to wrap around her waist. Some sonographers prefer the patient to sit at the end of the examination couch and then raise the patient's legs on a chair, others put the patient's legs in stirrups (1x) and some use an ultrasound pelvic pad (1w & 1y).

When the pelvis is not elevated during a TV scan, it becomes difficult if not impossible to see and have access to the ovaries and the urethra may be mistaken for a mass. It is paramount that, at all times, sonographers scan at the right height for them and that they maintain an appropriate scanning posture so as to avoid wrist, shoulder and spine problems, which may be inevitable later in life for them if care is not taken.

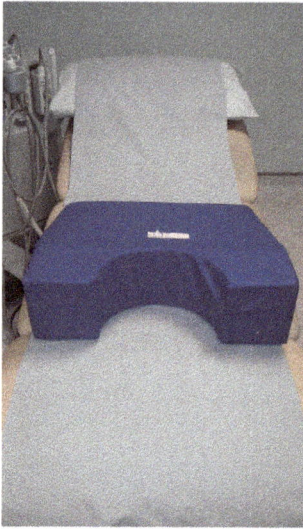 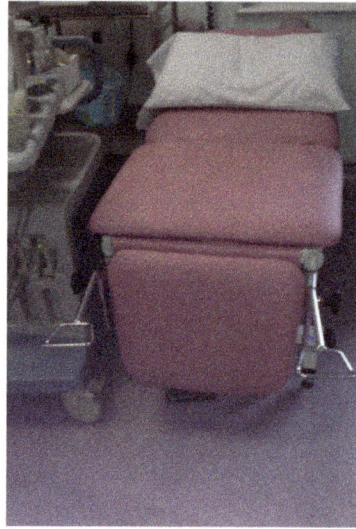

1w   **1x**

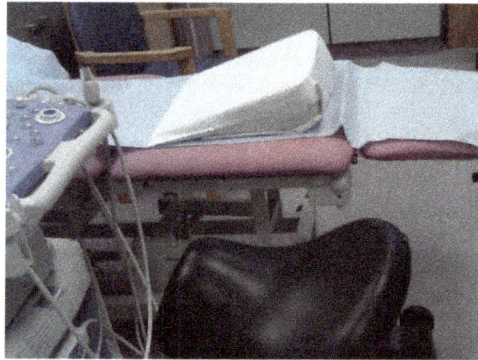

1y
Examples of ultrasound scanning couches with and without stirrups

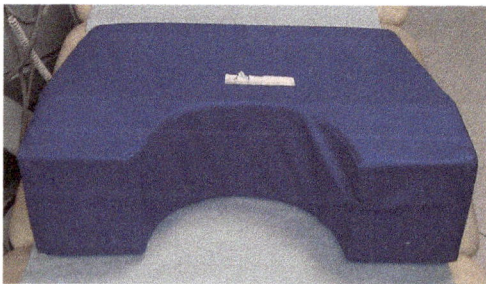 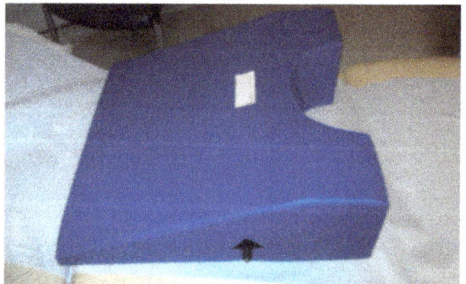

1z *An ultrasound scanning pad*   **1aa** *Lateral or side view*

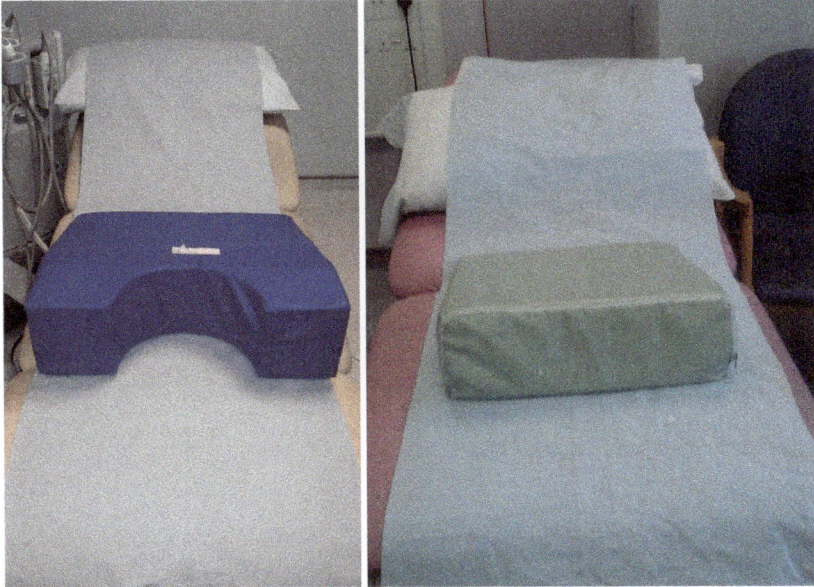

1ab   **1ac**
Two examples of transvaginal ultrasound scanning pads

A disposable incontinent pad should be used to cover the scanning pad before use and disposed of after each patient has been scanned.

The examination should be carried out with minimum discomfort to the patient. Care and gentleness should be applied when inserting the trans-vaginal probe, when moving the probe to obtain the necessary views and when removing the probe. It is advisable to carry out the examination and carefully document it before offering to show or point out the findings on the TV screen especially when the news is bad.

The TV probe should not be removed before discussing the findings with the patient, especially if the news is bad, as the patient or couple may wish to see what the bad news is about. For good or bad news, it is a prudent practice for the ultrasonographer to offer to show the patient and her husband or partner the ultrasound findings on the TV screen before gently removing the TV probe. The patient and her husband or partner's wishes should be respected should she or they decline this offer.

In many units, patients may purchase copies of the baby's pictures with a small donation or a token for this. When the news is bad, the patient is offered the picture(s) free of charge and any donation or money paid for the token is refunded to her. A hardcopy of the pregnancy image should be offered to the patient in a sealed envelope in case she may need it later. If she refuses the hardcopy, then it should be filed in her notes – just in case she wants it in the future. The patient's/couple wishes are to be respected at all times.

Following the examination, the patient should be offered some wipes to clean herself and be allowed her privacy as she gets dressed.

Sale of ultrasound pictures

This a long-established practice in many hospitals in the United Kingdom where a patient or her partner might want to have copies of the scan pictures of their expected baby or babies. Whether patients should pay an agreed price for these pictures or make a donation, should be clearly defined in the hospital's policies and procedures, which should be displayed in the patients' waiting area and ultrasound room. Should such funds be kept in the scanning room? It is not unusual to have coin-taking and ticket or token giving machines in the patients' waiting/reception area for those who wish to obtain copies of their ultrasound pictures. This course of action relieves the sonographer of much stress and danger. Hospital policies and procedures should also decide who periodically collects the money, who will be handling this money and what the money is used for.

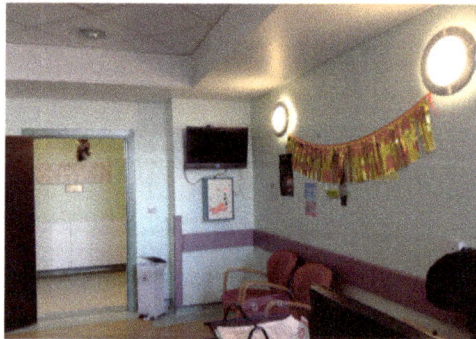

1ad
*An example of a coin-taking and token giving machine in a
patients' waiting or reception area*

Reporting package

It is better to use an agreed computerised reporting package so that reports are

standardised, each ultrasound report should include the following information:
- Hospital details
- Patients' details
- LMP if or where known
- Clinical indications for the scan
- Ultrasound findings, e.g. number of IUGS, YS, embryonic or fetal pole and CRL, the integrity of the sac, sac(s) and the presence of EHBs or FHBs and movements or otherwise
- GSD or GSV or CRL
- GA and EDD
- Assessment of the ovaries
- Assessment of the adnexa and POD
- Ultrasound impression or conclusion
- Any need for follow-up – when, why and where?
- Date of the ultrasound scan
- Name of the ultrasonographer
- Name and designation of chaperone, if used

Safety considerations

There are many safety issues that sonographers need to be aware of. They need to take the necessary actions to make every single examination safe for patients, relatives, themself and their colleagues. When an accident occurs in the department, it has to be documented, reported, investigated and reviewed so that any recommended changes can be effected to prevent such events reoccurring.

Biological safety

Many patients who attend the EGU for pregnancy complications come in the first trimester: a period of organogenesis which is known to be particularly sensitive to external influences.

According to the AIUM (1988) there is no evidence of biological effects from ultrasound on patients at intensities typical of instruments in current use. Nevertheless, prudent diagnostic ultrasound examinations should involve the use of minimum output levels and exposure times. In 1996, the European Federation of Societies for Ultrasound in Medicine and Biology (EFSUMB) recommended that until further scientific information is available, investigations using Doppler ultrasound at maximum output levels (in which the embryo (fetus) lies within the ultrasonic beam) be considered unadvisable. The sonographer should depending on where he is, practise within the set standards of organisations, including the British Medical Ultrasound Society (BMUS) or American Institute of Ultrasound in Medicine (AIUM) and the World Federation of Ultrasound in Medicine and Biology (WFUMB).

Sonographers are responsible for providing a safe and accurate ultrasound service. Furthermore, they should make regular improvements in their techniques and keep up to date with the current developments in their profession.

Sonographers can curtail the patient level ultrasound dose by taking the following precautions - not in any particular order :

- Ensuring good patient preparation
- Not performing unnecessary scans
- Ensuring that only qualified personnel scan
- Ensuring correct patient identification prior to the examination
- Carefully interpreting the clinical history and examination request
- Ensuring that the patient understands what the examination entails and consents to it
- Using the lowest possible output power (ALARA) (as low as reasonable achievable because of the potential for tissue heating when the thermal index exceeds 1) consistent with good quality images
- Removing the transducer from contact with the patient's skin when the Sonographer is not actually scanning
- Students training in ultrasound should do so under qualified supervision
- Performing regular equipment maintenance so that optimum operating levels are ensured
- Knowing the pregnancy test result ([ß]beta-HCG) level pre-scan will help ensure that the examination is tailored appropriately

Infection control

Every part of the ultrasound equipment needs to be cleaned regularly in line with the manufacturer's instructions. Particular attention needs to be focused on the cleanliness of the TA and TV probes and their cables. At the end of each examination, the gel should first be wiped off the TA probe with a dry wipe and then cleaned with wet wipes that are suitable for the equipment, e.g. use of Clinell wipes and other recommended wipes or the manufacturer's recommended cleaning wipes. The need to pay particular attention to the cleanliness of the TV probe cannot be over - emphasised. Suitable probe covers must be used for each examination and disposed off at the end of each examination. At the end of a TV examination, a visual check should be made to ensure that, during the examination, no split has occurred in the probe cover before disposing of it.

It is a good practice to clean the probe before putting it back in its holder. In addition to the routine cleaning, there might be need for disinfection or sterilisation of the ultrasound probe.(See an example of a sterilization process below).

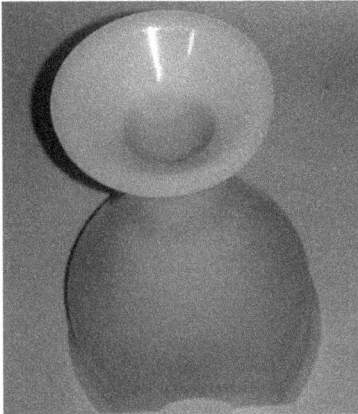 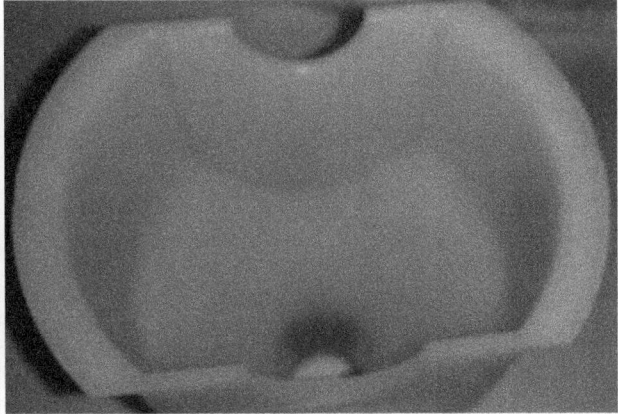

1ae   1af

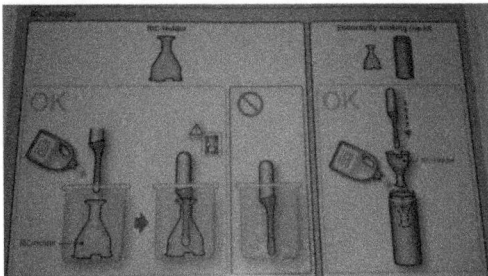

1ag

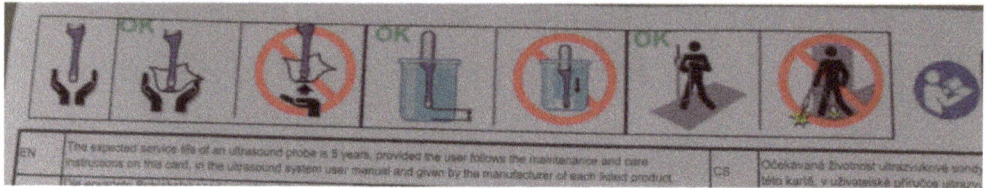

1ah
Example of the trans-vaginal probe sterilisation process/ technique.
(Used with the permission of GE Healthcare)

Sonographers can limit cross contamination by paying attention to the following:

- Good hand washing practice between patients. It is good practice to ensure that hand-washing and equipment cleaning are carried out at the commencement of and the completion of each TV scan examination as this will reassure the patient that effective infection control measures have been used

- Using a high level disinfection process combined with the use of a sterile gel and transducer covers as recommended by the manufacturer's instruction

- Ensuring that all the scanning sundries are within easy reach on a nearby trolley.

- Taking care not to use any probe cover that has a split in it

- Ensuring that probes do not have cracks, tears or abrasions which may harbour potential contaminants, thus leading to cross infection

- Making sure that, sonographers who wear gloves in both hands and make use of the other hand to help in the insertion of the TV probe, remove this glove before they commence the ultrasound examination and document the results of the scan. Otherwise using the soiled hand to operate the keyboard on the ultrasound equipment may introduce all forms of infection on the equipment – the spread of which might become uncontrollable

- Recording correctly the time, date, disinfection methods and verification of the results of the disinfectant's effectiveness

- Covering ultrasound scanning pads (where used) with an incontinent sheet to avoid the deposit of body fluids (see below). Such pads should be wiped clean at regular intervals, the incontinent sheet changed after each patient and the scanning pad is stored not on the floor, but perhaps on a shelf or in a dedicated holder (see below)

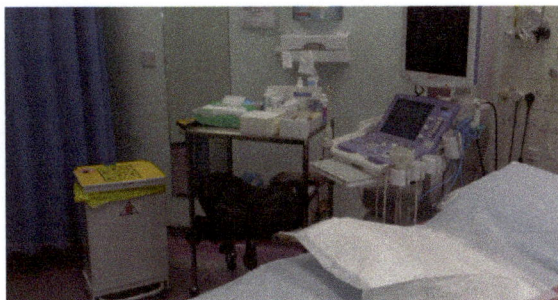

1ai
Incontinent sheet over the scanning pad

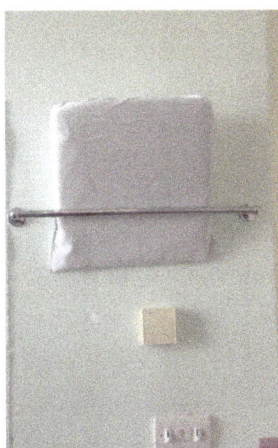 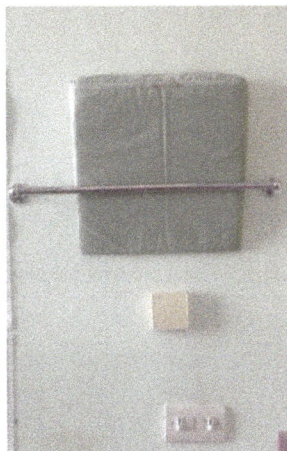

1aj   **1ak**
Dedicated scanning pad holders

Physical safety of the sonographer, patients and relatives

Ultrasound examinations are carried out under dim lighting. There are cables for the ultrasound equipment, the couch, and the gel bottle warmer. It is essential that the physical safety of the sonographer, patients and relatives should be considered and addressed. To enhance the physical safety of all it is advisable to adhere to the following suggestions (not in any particular order):

- Ensure that there is a clear pathway for sonographers in the ultrasound room for their work
- Ensure that the layout or arrangement of the ultrasound accessories and other furniture do not have the cables running on the floor where anyone can trip over them
- Ensure there is a clear pathway for patients and their relatives
- Room lighting should be at a level suitable to the patient's eye so that there is

ease of clear movement
- Ultrasound couches should be lowered or adjusted to the patient's individual level so that it is easy for the patient to get to and from the couch before and after the scan
- Sonographers should remove the scanning pad (where and when used) at the end of the TVS before the patient is asked to come off the couch
- Assistance should be offered and given when and where possible to patients who might need it in their getting on and down from the scanning couch
- Postmenopausal patients who come for emergency gynaecology scan and may be prone to dizziness should be allowed to sit up first and given some time to get their balance before standing up after a procedure
- It is safer to have the room lights undimmed when the patient is getting from the ultrasound couch
- Liquid spills are to be avoided and all spills are to be cleaned to avoid anyone slipping in the ultrasound room
- Babies and toddlers are to be secured in their buggies and given the appropriate snack or toy before the commencement of the examination or supervised by the accompanying adult to prevent them from running around in the ultrasound room during the patient's ultrasound examination
- Mothers, whilst on the examination couch, should have no need to stretch in order to calm a crying child
- There should be normal lighting in the toilet suite for patients
- Falls or injuries, involving either staff, patients or relatives in the ultrasound room or patients' toilet are to be reported and documented as per hospital protocol
- Following a fall or injury the person who fell or is injured should be seen by a doctor or unit nurse and treated if and where possible before they leave the ultrasound unit
- The incidence of documented physical falls should be reviewed and lessons learnt from these accidents and recommendations should be quickly put in force in order to prevent other falls
- The ultrasound room should be devoid of all unwanted or un-needed stock or furniture. In other words, the ultrasound room should not be made the storage place for unwanted furniture items
- Having a separate small storeroom for ultrasound accessories such as gels

and blue rolls will make the room easier to tidy up and provide more free space in the scanning room

- Instructions about changing pre- or post-TVS should be made clear and simple to avoid falls
- Ultrasound scanning couch height should be made clear to the patient pre- and post-TVS
- The emergency call out button or switch must be within an easy access for the Sonographer.
- Extra care is to be taken where a patient will have to be transferred from a wheelchair or stretcher onto the ultrasound couch and vice versa
- Each sonographer must comply with the hospital's training policy on Safe Manual Handling and CPR (Cardiopulmonary resuscitation) amongst others policies
- Sonographers must be very vigilant, especially when giving 'bad news' to a couple as occasionally it is the husband or partner who unknowingly breaks down or is at an increased risk of falling on the floor and should be rescued and supported before he lands on the floor
- Safe manual handling techniques, appropriate for the situation, should be used if and when needed
- Agreed written policies or guidelines or pathways should be available on what to do when there is a physical injury involving a patient, relative or member of staff in the EPAGU
- Sonographers are at risk of tripping over cables that are left dangling on the floor and not properly put in the hooks on the machines. Therefore, all probes or equipment cables should be put in the place where they belong
- Should the sonographer decide to sit on a scanning stool with castor wheels then he must sit properly on the stool and put his feet on the floor to prevent unwanted sliding on the floor of the ultrasound room

Electrical and physical safety of the equipment

The expected life span of an ultrasound probe is 5 years, provided the user follows the maintenance and care instructions given by the manufacturer. Non-hazardous voltage is present during normal transducer or probe use. Regular electrical safety leakage testing is recommended to ensure operator and equipment safety. Cables should be checked daily and routinely for cuts, tears, and kinking. The TA & TVS probes should be checked for damage and the television monitors checked.

When any probe is showing signs of magnetic drop-out (see 1al), it needs repair or replacement so that shadows from the drop-out do not obscure any vital information whilst scanning.

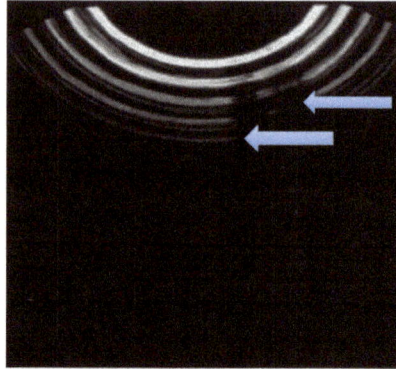

1al
An example of fall out or drop-out in a TV probe (arrows)

Sonographers' safety

Sonographers are prone to work-related musculoskeletal disorders (WRMSD and repetitive strain injury RSI) due to factors such as increased patient referrals, increasing BMI in the population and scanning in a wrong posture. To prevent or limit WRMSD, hospitals should adhere to the following recommendations:

- Provide equipments that are fit for purpose, e.g. a couch and scanning chair with height adjustable facilities
- Provide a 'power grip' to hold the transducer
- Provide separate viewing monitors for the sonographer and the patient
- Avoid overcrowding the sonographer's list. When and where there is a trainee in attendance, the allocated time given should be such that there is an adequate time to perform the examination of the patient and provide the required teaching of the trainee
- Make provision in the rota for the sonographer to have short but frequent breaks from scanning
- Ensure that the sonographer is not asked to repeatedly carry out the same type of scanning examination

Sonographers should ensure that provisions are made for the following necessities

- Setting the room temperature including the air-conditioning to a comfortable level at the beginning of their sessions (am or pm)
- Adjusting the room light to suitable levels for both examination and report writing
- Keeping healthy as much as it is practicable
- Placing their feet flat on the ground when sitting down to scan
- Exercising and stretching before starting to scan and in between patients
- Using the provided 'power grip' to hold the transducer rather than a finger (pinch) grip
- Having all the scanning sundries within easy reach on a nearby trolley
- Abduction the scanning arm to the least possible angle by positioning the patient appropriately on the couch
- Using correct positioning whilst they are scanning
- Varying their scanning position during the examination
- Taking short but frequent breaks from scanning so they can stretch, have a drink, visit the toilet
- Taking responsibility for addressing personal workload issues, e.g. stress-related issues following communicating bad news

Quality issues

Scanning set-ups should consider the following:
- Sonographer's experience and limitations
- Perhaps the need for more sonographers
- High standard precision equipment with good resolution, playback or cine-loop facility and TV probes
- Legal implications for sonographers communicating ultrasound examination results
- Access to other departments should the patient need further investigations, e.g. MRI or CT in a diagnostic imaging department, laboratory for further laboratory tests
- Access to a fetal medicine unit within the hospital or referral centre where the hospital does not have any in case of the need for invasive testing or second level scan as and when required

- Programme for a continuous audit of work

Realities
- Are there any additional training needs?
- Will there be the provision of chaperones for same sex examinations?
- What sort of service will the unit be providing and can patients self-refer?
- Range of techniques and the ultrasound services provided
- Cost implications – space, room, equipment, staff cost, cost-effectiveness of service
- Cost implications – initial set-up and running costs
- Administrative aspects – separate dedicated administrative staff or use of ANC or radiology or EPAGU administrative staff, filing systems and other considerations
- Staffing – sonographers from the radiology department or newly appointed and dedicated sonographers for the new unit
- Sonographers' annual leave, sick leave, study-day leave and the implicated costs
- Will the ultrasound equipment be used ten sessions per week? If not, for what percentage of time will the ultrasound equipment be left unused? (a session being half a day, i.e. a.m. or p.m.)

Benefits of having a dedicated ultrasound unit in EPAGU
- Patients are in a better, more relaxed environment with facilities for privacy, unlike the A&E department
- Patients, family and friends are no longer exposed to ill patients in the radiology department, nor seen in an X-ray or radiation environment
- Patients are not exposed to happy pregnant patients in the ANC
- With the EPAGU being a consultant-led unit, it is now easier and less stressful for the patient to be seen and assessed by an obstetrician and gynaecologist or midwife, especially when there is bad news
- Patients are given professional care by a specialist team of doctors, midwives and sonographers
- It may be easier to organise a one-stop clinic for patients, especially for those who need follow-ups
- Patients are seen sooner than they would be if scanned in the main

ultrasound unit or radiology unit
- Direct access for patients from GPs, other consultants in the hospital and from A&E doctors
- Patients are seen sooner than they would be seen amongst others in an A&E department
- Reduction in hospital bed usage as diagnoses can be made quicker and most patients do not require hospital beds for many conditions
- GPs can get feedback much quicker
- A dedicated scanning unit helps with the 4-hour A&E target/waiting times
- Unlike the A&E department, patients in EPAGU are cared for in an environment that provides for their privacy needs
- Dedicated and trained Sonographer and scanning facilities with results available immediately after each scan.

After the new set-up – what next?
- Evaluating the new or refurbished set-up by conducting surveys – simply by observing the comments of staff, patients or relatives or
- Conducting questionnaire surveys

As the new set-up is evaluated, there might be need for minor changes; however, one should not lose hope or feel repulsed.

There is also the need to have regular team meetings where experience and good practices could be shared and a place to learn.

Chapter Conclusion

Having a dedicated EPAGU with ultrasound facilities can be rewarding especially for patients, but the facility needs to be carefully thought through, planned, executed, managed and regularly evaluated.

Bibliography Chapter 1

Book:

Deane CR. (2011) Practical Ultrasound – Using Scanner and Optimizing Ultrasound Images. In: Clinical Ultrasound. Volume 1. (Chapter 3). 3rd ed. Allan PL, Baxter GM and Weston MJ. (editors). Edinburgh. Elsevier Churchill Livingstone.

Articles:
Arthritis Research UK (2013) Shoulder Pain. Available at: http://www.arthritisresearchuk.org/arthritis-information/conditions/shoulder-pain.aspx

Baby Scan Home Videos should be Stopped. Ultrasound SOR News. Synergy news, August 2010. www.sor.org/ http:/www.bbc_radio_five_live.

Bly S, Van Den Hof MC. Obstetric Ultrasound Biological Effects and Safety. J Obstet Gynaecol Can. 2005 Jun 27(6):572–580. Available at: www.ncbi.nlm.nih.gov/pubmed/16100635

Bottomley F. (2008) Ultrasound Safety: A Sonographer's Viewpoint. BMUS, HEAUltrasound 16(4):238.

The new British Medical Ultrasound Society Guidelines for the safe use of diagnostic ultrasound equipment
Gail ter Haar. Available at:

http://journals.sagepub.com/doi/full/10.1258/ult.2010.100007

Brown TG. (2011 August) Repetitive Strain Injuries: would it help if Sonographers Could Work Facing Across the Couch and Patient, instead of Parallel to Them? Ultrasound 19(3):178–179.

Department of Health (2013) Maternity Care Facilities: Planning and Design (HBN 09–02) Available at: https://www.gov.uk/government/publications/guidance-for-the-planning-and-design-of-maternity-care-facilities.
(See sections on ultrasound services and early pregnancy care.)

Department of Health (2001) HBN 6: Volume 1, Facilities for Diagnostic Imaging and Interventional Radiology. Available at: https://www.gov.uk/government/publications/facilities-for-diagnostic-imaging-and-interventional-radiology. (See section on ultrasound imaging (p.101.)

Department of Veterans Affairs – Radiology Service Design Guide (Ultrasound Room (XDUS1) April 2008. https://www.wbdg.org/ccb/VA/VADEGUID/radio.pdf

GE Healthcare (2014) Ultrasound Transducers. Available at: http://www3.gehealthcare.com/en/products/categories/ultrasound/ultrasound_probes. (Recommended care and handling procedures for ultrasound transducers.)

Gibbs V, Young P. Methods to prevent or reduce work-related musculoskeletal disorders amongst sonographers. Synergy. July 2011. [availabe: print copy, British Library, (P) GQ20-E(65)]

Gibbs V & Young P. (2008) Work-related Musculoskeletal Disorders in Sonography and the Alexander Technique. BMUS, Ultrasound 16(4):213–219.

Gregory V. Musculoskeletal Injuries: An Occupational Health And Safety Issue in Sonography. Available at: https://mail.soundergo.com/pdf/mskarticle.pdf

Guidance on Ultrasound Procedures in Early Pregnancy (1995). Royal College of Radiologists.
Guidelines for Professional Working Standards Ultrasound Practice United Kingdom Association of Sonographers. October 2008.

Health Building Note 09–02. Maternity Care Facilities. Ultrasound Suite. Available at: www.gov.uk/government upload/system.

Hides J. HSE Sonography Report. Column 25, 1. 2013. pp. 14–19. Work-related Musculoskeletal Injuries in Sonographers – Why are sonographers wearing out? Available at: www.hse.gov.uk/heathservices/management-of-musculoskeletal-disorders-in-sonography-work.pdf.

Monnington SC, Dodd-Hughes K, Milnes E, Ahmad Y (2012) Risk Management of Musculoskeletal Disorders in Sonography Work. HSE Corporate Science, Engineering and Analysis Directorate Project Report. Available at: http://www.hse.gov.uk/healthservices/management-of-musculoskeletal – disorders-in-sonography-work.pdf

Monnington SC, Dodd-Hughes K, Milnes E, Ahmad Y. HSE Corporate Science, Engineering and Analysis Directorate Project Report – Risk Management of Musculoskeletal Disorders in Sonography. 23 March 2012.
Available at: http://www.hse.gov.uk/msd/index.htm

Morgan MA, Gaillard F, et al. Early pregnancy. Available at http://radiopaedia. org/articles/early_pregnancy.

Murphy C, Russo A. (2000) An Update on Ergonomic Issues in Sonography. Available at: https://www.sdms.org/pdf/sonoergonomics.pdf

Preventing Occupational Injury Among Diagnostic Medical Sonographers. Available at: https://www.sdms.org/pdf/preventinginjury.pdf

Royal College of Radiologists & Royal College of Obstetricians and Gynaecologists (1995) Guidance on Ultrasound Procedures in Early Pregnancy. RCR Ref. No BFCR (95)B.

Society of Radiographers. General Guidelines. Available at: http://www.sor.org/ learning/document-library/guidelines-professional-working-standards

Sonography work in healthcare. (2013) Available at: http://www.hse.gov.uk/ healthservices/sonography-work-in-healthcare.htm

Thomson N (2015) Sale of Images, Determination of Fetal Sex and Commercial Aspects Related to NHS Obstetric Ultrasound Examinations. 2nd ed. Available at: http://www.sor.org/learning/document-library/sale-images-determination-fetal-sex-and-commercial-aspects-related-nhs-obstetric-ultrasound-6

Thomson N (2015) Standards for the Provision of an Ultrasound Service. Available at: http://www.sor.org/sites/default/files/document versions/ bfcr1417_standards_ultrasound.pdf

Thomson N (2014) Work Related Musculoskeletal Disorders (Sonographers). Available at: http://www.sor.org/learning/document-library/work-related-musculo-skeletal-disorders-sonographers

Thomson N, Wigley L. The Management and Prevention of Work-related Musculoskeletal Disorders. Synergy news. December 2011. [available: print copy, British Library, (P) GP41 (R) – E(2)]

United Kingdom Association of Sonographers (2008) Guidelines for Professional Working Standards Ultrasound Practice. Available at: http://www.sor.org/ learning/document-library/guidelines-professional-working-standards-ultrasound-practice

Wigley L. Protecting the Sonography. Synergy news. November 2011. [available: print copy, British Library, 8585. 934850]

www.spaceforhealth.nhs.uk/articles/pregnancy-fetal-and – maternal – assessment-uk.

www.spaceforhealth.nhs.uk/articles/ultrasound-suite.

www.spaceforhealth.nhs.uk/articles/diagnostic – facilities.

www.spaceforhealth.nhs.uk/articles/early-pregnancy-assessment – unit.

www.spaceforhealth.nhs.uk/articles/spaces-7

www/sor.org/learning/document-library/guidelines-professional-working-standards.

Young P, Gibbs V. Is the Alexander Technique the Answer? Synergy. March 2009. [available: print copy, British Library, (P) GQ20-E(65)]

Chapter 2

Normal first trimester ultrasound appearances

- Normal first trimester ultrasound appearances
- Pregnancy dating in the first trimester
- Assisted conception
- Ultrasound examination reporting
- Ultrasound identifiable anatomy in the first trimester
- Maternal ovaries in pregnancy
- Corpus luteum
- Luteal phase defect
- Follicle or corpus luteal cyst
- Measurements in early pregnancy
- Yolk sac
- Vitelline duct
- Amniotic fluid
- Documenting EHB or FHB (bpm)

Normal first trimester ultrasound appearances

High-resolution ultrasonography and trans-vaginal ultrasound techniques have resulted in enhanced visualisation of embryonic and extra-embryonic structures. The resolution of the ultrasound equipment, real-time scanning or imaging, the knowledge and the experience of the sonographer mean that it is possible to identify normal and some abnormal structures in the maturing embryo or fetus. It must be stressed, however, that acquiring these ultrasound images and their interpretation is very much dependent on the sonographer performing the ultrasound examination.

It is essential that the sonographer be familiar with the normal ultrasound appearances of a growing embryo or fetus in order to be able to relate the findings with the clinical history, the gestational age (GA) of the pregnancy; and, make a diagnosis.

A good knowledge of anatomy and embryology is important because of the rapid growth and changes in ultrasound appearances, especially in the first trimester of pregnancy because then it will be easier to identify any abnormal anatomy and avoid potential pitfalls. The ovaries and the adnexa should be checked and documentation of ultrasound findings is essential when performing early pregnancy scans.

Pregnancy dating in the first trimester

This is done by using any of the following methods:
Gestational sac volume (GSV) or gestational sac diameter (GSD) – used when the embryonic pole is not yet seen or measurable.

The gestational sac size, yolk sac (YS) size and embryonic or fetal pole measurements should be considered together, and they should correspond to each other for a diagnosis of a normal or abnormal pregnancy; dates will be established later.

Crown rump length (CRL) (+/- 4.7 days) (Robinson & Flemming 1975). This is used when the embryonic/fetal pole is measurable to about 13+6 weeks or a CRL of up to 84mm. From 14/40, the head circumference (HC), biparietal diameter (BPD) and femur length (FL) are the measurements usually used.

Every gestation begins as a single cell, but eventually individual differences in growth rate give rise to a range of sizes, all of which are normal for a given GA. Early in the pregnancy these individual differences are much less pronounced than they are later; therefore, correct dating is more reliable.

Measurements correctly done in the first trimester are more dependable than those done later in the pregnancy.

This patient was referred for a dating scan with a clinical history of unknown LMP. Both ovaries (not shown here) appeared sonographically normal.

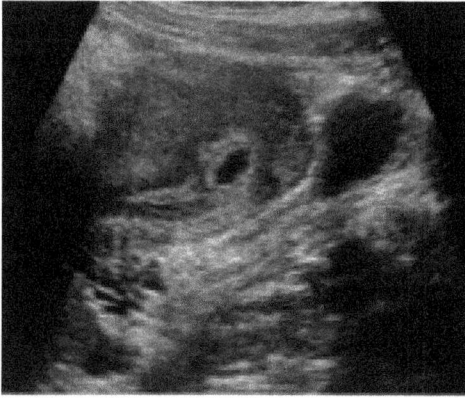

2.1a *Longitudinal section (LS)*   **2.1b**   *Transverse section (TS)*

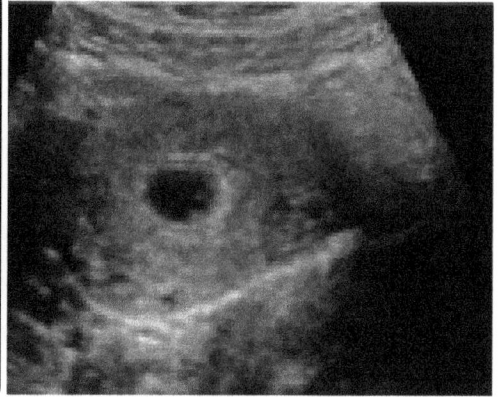

Trans-abdominal scan view (TAS) showing an anteverted uterus (A/V) uterus with an intrauterine gestational sac (IUGS). The YS is hardly visible.

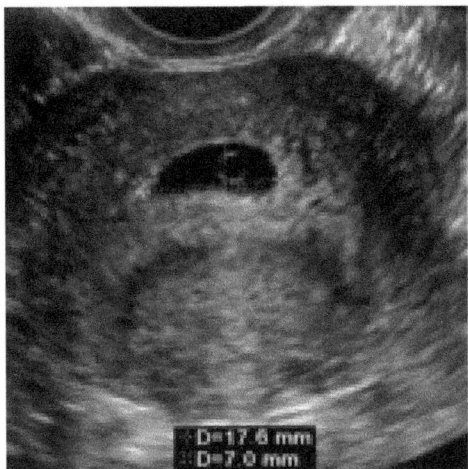

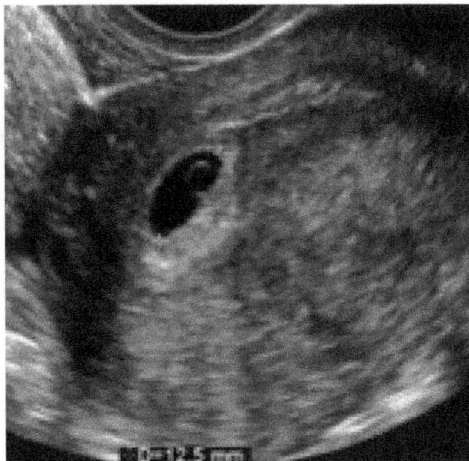

2.1c   **TS**   **2.1d - LS** *measuring the GS*

The same patient: note the resolution between TAS and trans-vaginal scan (TVS). Images for this patient are a few minutes apart from each other.

There are reporting packages that will work out the GA from the above GS measurement. Alternatively, we calculate the GSV using the formula – (anteroposterior (AP) × longitudinal × transverse diameter) cm × 0.5233= ml. In the above example that will be: 1.25 × 1.76 × 0.7 × 0.5233 = 0.8ml. Using the appropriate chart in the unit, the GA of this pregnancy is 5+1/40.

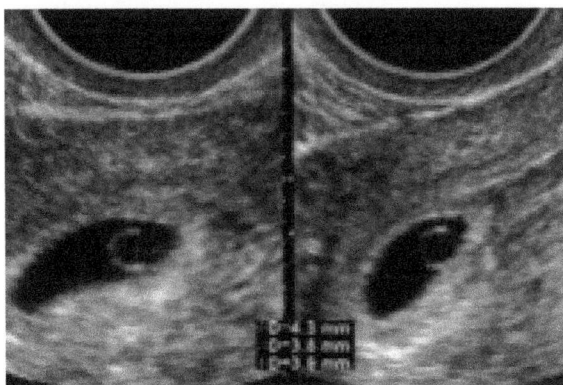

2.1e
Trans-vaginal scan views of the same patient
(Showing the IUGS and the YS measured.)

The YS has been measured above. Some reporting packages can use the YS measurements to date the early pregnancy before the EMP becomes visible.

Ultrasound findings: An IUGS with a YS. No EP is demonstrated. YS measured 4.3 × 3.8 × 3.9mm.

Impression: An intrauterine pregnancy (IUP). Perhaps too early to visualise the EMP.

However, where a patient does not have any other medical complaints such as pains that might be related to the pregnancy, the sonographer should suggest a follow-up dating scan in 2–3 weeks from this scan to confirm that the pregnancy is ongoing or otherwise. In addition, the review scan may show the number of heartbeats present and can date the pregnancy more accurately as the CRL will be measurable by then in a normal ongoing pregnancy.

Dating may be the reason for performing an early ultrasound examination, but it is not uncommon to find unexpected findings (not in this case), which may need to be addressed then or later in the pregnancy.

Assisted conception

For most, if not all assisted conceptions, it is a standard practice that the patient will have been given an expected date of delivery (EDD) at the time of the success of her treatment. However, if and where she has not been given this and the sonographer has to assign an EDD based on the fertility treatment, here is how to calculate the LMP:

Frozen Embryo transfer (FET) – Establish from the patient the embryo transfer date, e.g. 18/01/2018. Establish also how old the embryo was at the time of the transfer, e.g. third day or fifth day transfer.

For day 3 embryo transfer – subtract 17 days from the embryo transfer date. LMP = 18/01/2018 – 17 days = 02/01/2018

For day 5 embryo transfer – subtract 19 days from the embryo transfer date. LMP = 18/01/2018 – 19 days = 31/12/2017

The sonographer can now use the calculated date as a normal LMP date.

GIFT/ICSI/IVF – To obtain an LMP in these patients, establish from the patient the day of the egg collection/retrieval. Use that date as day 15 of the cycle and use that to recalculate the LMP. So, if the egg collection date is 22/12/2017, then the LMP = 22/12/2017 – 15 days = 08/12/2017.

Ultrasound examination reporting

Immediately following the ultrasound examination an ultrasound report should be generated containing the following information:

- Hospital details
- Patient's details
- LMP (if known)
- Date of scan
- Reason for scan or clinical history
- Answer to examination request
- Adjusted or corrected GA and EDD by ultrasound if indicated
- Ultrasound equipment used, e.g. Aloka, Toshiba
- Method of scanning (TAS or TVS)
- Quality of views obtained – good, poor or restricted and why?
- Any other important findings, such as the uterus, embryo or fetus, ovaries or the adnexa
- Any other relevant comments
- Any need for follow-up or suggestions
- Name of the sonographer (Only qualified sonographers should be allowed to provide the ultrasound report of the scan performed.)
- Trainee students will have to have their report countersigned by the sonographer supervising the examination.
- Any problems encountered during the examination should be documented, e.g. factors that make the examination limited either by the quality of the images obtained or the patient's discomfort or their declining to have a TVS where it is not contraindicated.
- Use of the appropriate obstetric graphs can help to simplify and clarify the ultrasound result to the patient and to the rest of the team. See Appendix 1 for such graphs.
- Technical challenges that the sonographer may encounter that may limit the quality of the ultrasound examination include:

- Patients' pain that limits the examination
- Shadows from pelvic masses and cysts
- Overlying bowel gas
- Very active bowels
- Retroverted and retroflexed uterus
- High body mass index (BMI)
- Embryo or fetus that is not in a favourable position in the maternal pelvis at the time of the scan.

Follow-up scans

It is not unusual for the sonographer or clinician to recommend a follow-up scan when:

- The GSD is less than 25mm
- Vaginal bleeding is not stopping
- The initial scan result is inconclusive
- Pregnancy is of unknown location (PUL)
- The CRL is less than 7mm without a FHB
- A CRL or heartbeat cannot be established as in 2.1a–e above
- Adnexal or ovarian cyst(s) with suspicious ultrasound features
- There is evidence of ovarian hyperstimulation syndrome (OHSS)
- Bizarre or unusual ultrasound findings that cannot be initially classified
- The pregnancy cannot be dated due to no embryonic pole yet or non measurable CRL
- Type of multiple pregnancies is yet to be established:DCDA or MCDA or MCMA
- There is negative suspicion of the ultrasound features, e.g. abnormal heartbeats that are slow or too fast
- It is essential that the previous ultrasound report and images be available at the follow-up appointment for sonographers to compare with their current findings. This can be through linked set-ups such as PACS or an ordinary standard report and images in the patient's file or notes

Ultrasound identifiable embryonic or fetal anatomy in the first trimester

This section of the book will focus on the observable normal anatomy on ultrasound in the first trimester. In addition to what is stated in this section, the study of any good book on embryology is advised and will be beneficial to the reader.

In a normal IUP, the first ultrasound identifiable evidence is a gestational sac. Prior to this, usually a thickened endometrium is seen which cannot be used as the yardstick for confirming an IUP. A thickened endometrium cannot be used to confirm, date or assess a pregnancy because the same appearance:

Is seen just before menstruation (late phase of the menstrual cycle)

Is seen as a decidual reaction that can be associated with ectopic pregnancy

Can be confused with RPOC

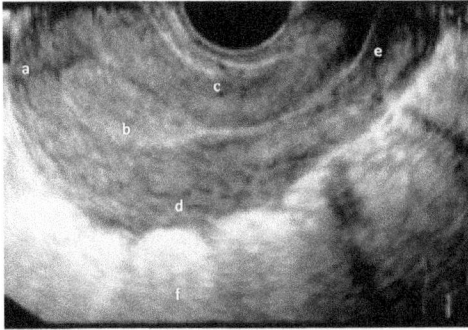

2.2a

a – fundal myometrium, b – endometrium, c – anterior myometrium
d- posterior myometrium, e – cervix, f – overlying bowel gas

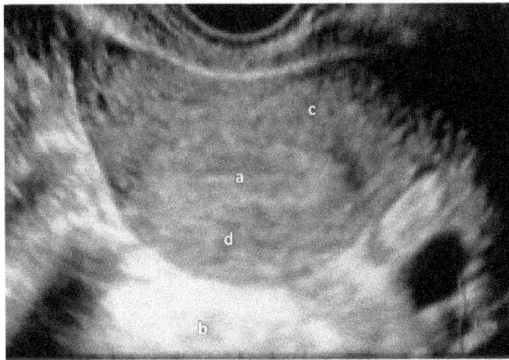

2.2b

a – endometrium b – overlying bowel gas, c – anterior myometrium,
d – posterior myometrium

The above was done for a patient who had a positive pregnancy test result at 6/40. Note there is no obvious IUGS demonstrated, but a thickened endometrium (a in

2.2a – 2.2b). Note the bowel gas posterior to the uterus (f in 2.2a & b in 2.2b). A thickened endometrium is essential for the implantation of the fertilised egg in the uterus.

In a normal ongoing pregnancy, some days later a small gestational sac will be seen and some days later the YS; then the pulsating fetal heart beats, then the embryonic pole. At the initial stages, the embryonic pole is always next to the YS (diamond ring sign).

Thickened endometrium --> GS, --> GS+YS, --> GS +YS + EHB,--> GS +YS+ EHB + EMP -> measurable CRL.

It is believed that the process of prenatal development occurs in three main stages. The germinal stage is the first 2 weeks after conception (GA 2–4/40); the embryonic period is from the third week to the eighth week (GA 5–10/40); and from the ninth week until birth is the fetal period (GA 11–40). There is rapid development and growth within the first trimester. The following images show normal ultrasound appearances at various GA.

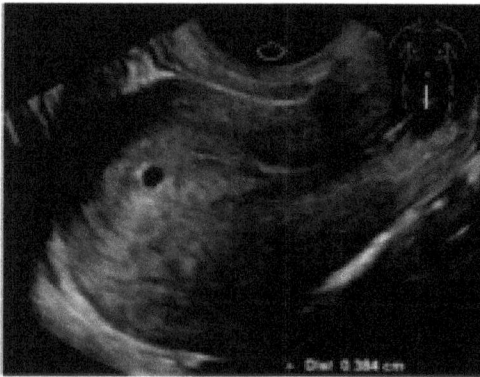

2.3a

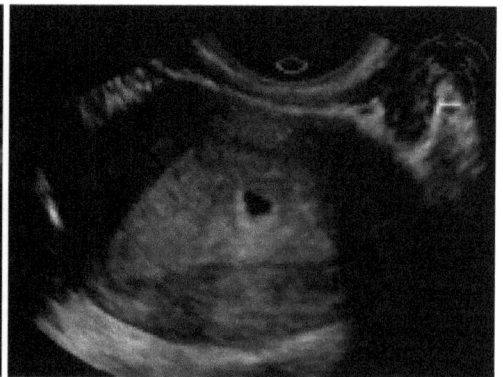

2.3b

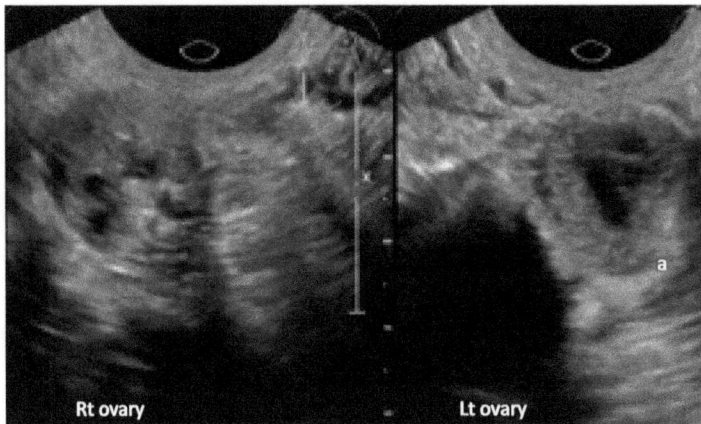

2.3c *a- corpus luteum in the left ovary*

Ultrasound findings: There is an approx. 0.4mm cystic entity in a thickened endometrium. This is probably an early intrauterine gestational sac (2.3 a–b). The right ovary appears sonographically normal. There is a corpus luteum in the left ovary (a), (2.3c), which is a normal finding at this stage of pregnancy.

Impression: Possibly a very early IUP.
A follow-up scan did confirm a singleton IUP.

Depending on the departmental protocol and the reason for the scan, if the above patient was scanned because of a suspected ectopic pregnancy and this was a natural conception, then a follow-up scan 7–10 days later will be suggested by the sonographer or referring clinician, provided the patient is asymptomatic or when the β-hCG result is high enough for an IUGS to be seen. If, on the other hand, she was scanned to check her dates and the patient does not have any symptoms of pain or vaginal bleeding, then her next scan would be a dating scan 3–4 weeks from the previous scan date. At the dating scan, a YS, measurable embryonic pole and EHB should be seen and the CRL measured provided the pregnancy, as expected, is ongoing.

Until the YS and EHB are seen, a single intrauterine gestational sac does not imply a singleton pregnancy.

Maternal ovaries in pregnancy

It is good practice to assess the patient's ovaries and adnexa, especially at the first scan in any pregnancy to confirm or exclude any abnormality or identify normal physiological changes in the ovaries or an adnexal mass that might have implications on the pregnancy. The findings should be documented in pictures and in writing as this will represent the baseline for any further follow-up scan.

Corpus luteum

The female egg grows in a sac called the follicle within the ovary. Once the egg is released from the follicle at ovulation in a natural cycle or at egg collection in an IVF/ICSI cycle, the remnant of the sac becomes the corpus luteum. This can be seen on ultrasound and with colour flow Doppler as it has the characteristic 'ring of fire appearance' (2.5b and 2.5c) The role of the corpus luteum is to produce progesterone which enables the endometrial lining to become thick for implantation and prevent shedding of the endometrium. Progesterone is produced by the corpus luteum until an approximate GA of 10 weeks when the placenta takes over until the end of the pregnancy. The developing embryo usually releases human chorionic gonadotropin (HCG), which encourages or stimulates the corpus luteum to keep producing progesterone.

Most women release a single egg in a natural unstimulated menstrual cycle; occasionally, they may release two. Seeing a corpus luteum on ultrasound in early pregnancy is a good sign and it indicates from which side the egg has been released. A small-sized corpus luteum generally does not cause problems and in the course of the pregnancy tends to disappear. Large cysts may make a patient prone to abdominal and/or pelvic pains, which can lead to torsion or rupture and ultimately to a visit to the emergency department. It is not uncommon to find a haemorrhagic corpus luteum, which on ultrasound is seen as fine interdigitating septations, a fishnet weave or fine reticular appearance within the cyst (2.5b). The location and size of the corpus luteum needs to be documented.

This patient was referred for a dating scan. She was unsure of her LMP.

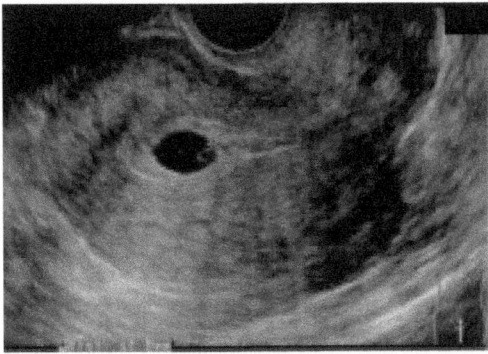

2.4a

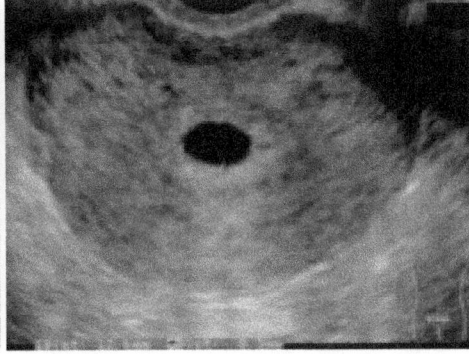

2.4b

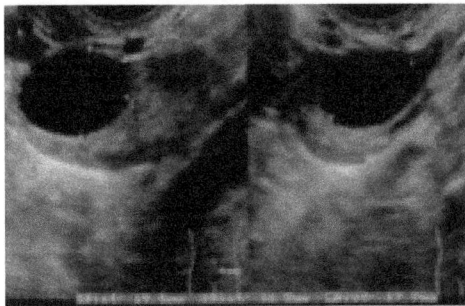

2.4c

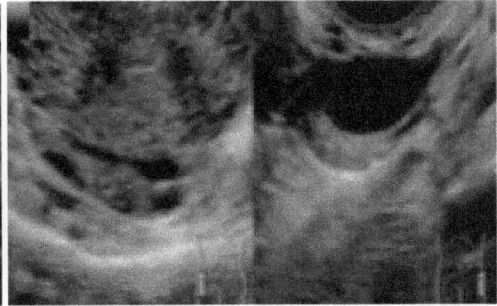

2.4d

Ultrasound findings: There is an IUGS measuring approx. 12 × 13 × 8mm (GSV = 1.2 × 1.3 × 0.8 × 0.5233 = 0.65ml) and a small YS. No embryonic pole is demonstrated. This is an early pregnancy (2.4a–b).

The right ovary appears sonographically normal. There is an approx. 19 × 16 × 18mm corpus luteum in the left ovary, which is a normal finding at this stage of pregnancy (2.4c–d).

Impression: A very early IUP and corpus luteum in the left ovary.

Until the embryonic pole and heartbeats are seen, it is unknown whether this will be a singleton or twin pregnancy – a monochorionic pregnancy (MC).

Luteal phase defect

Luteal phase defect occurs when the corpus luteum does not produce sufficient progesterone to sustain the pregnancy. This deficiency causes shedding of the endometrial lining thus leading to a miscarriage. It is important to document the presence or absence of a corpus luteum in early pregnancy and especially in patients who have had miscarriages or are having a miscarriage.

Follicle or corpus luteal cyst?

An ovarian follicle is a fluid-filled sac in which there is a growing oocyte or immature egg. Once the egg is matured and released at ovulation or at egg collection e.g. during IVF/ICSI treatment, the remant of the sac gets fluid filled and becomes a corpus luteal cyst. Though both are fluid filled, there are some differences in their ultrasound appearances.

Follicle	Corpus luteal cyst
Always round or circular, smooth outline	May be irregular in outline, not always round
Seen pre ovulation	Seen post ovulation
Never haemorrhagic and never have internal echoes	May become haemorrhagic and may have internal echoes
With Colour Doppler 'no ring of fire' appearance	With Colour Doppler will have 'ring of fire appearance'
No accompanying free pelvic fluid	Often seen with some accompanying free pelvic fluid
Normal follicle	Normal 'ring of fire' appearance
	Haemorrhagic corpus Luteum. Arrow shows some free fluid

Measurements in early pregnancy

The method of measuring or dating an early pregnancy will depend on the ultrasound findings. The thickness of the endometrium cannot be used as a means of dating the pregnancy for the reasons already mentioned earlier.

Until the embryonic or fetal pole is seen and can be measured and charted, the way to estimate the pregnancy is by measuring the gestational sac and using the GSV or GSD or YS charts.

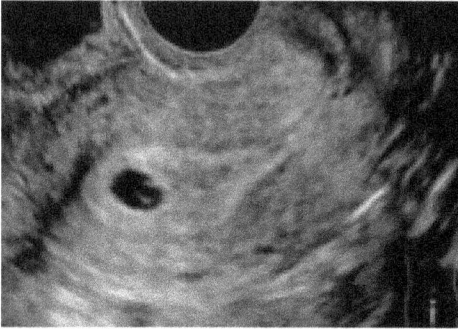

2.6a　IUGS +YS @ 5+5/40

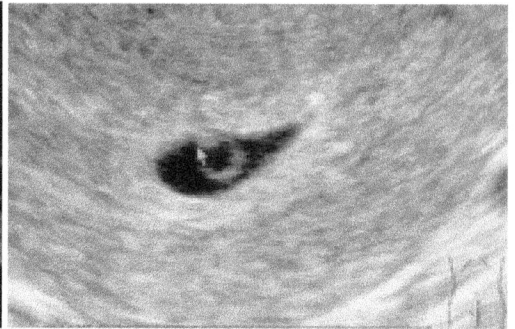

2.6b　CRL = 1.7mm. EHB seen

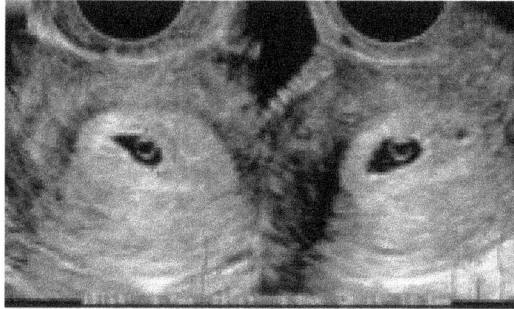

2.6c
GSV measurement @ 5+5 /40 = 0.67 × 0.65 × 1.13cm × 0.5233 = 0.29ml.

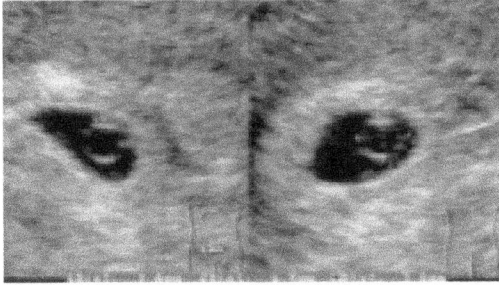

2.6d *YS measurement @ 5+5 /40 = 3.6 × 4.5 × 3.6mm*

Normal ultrasound appearances at various GA.

4 – 5+5/40

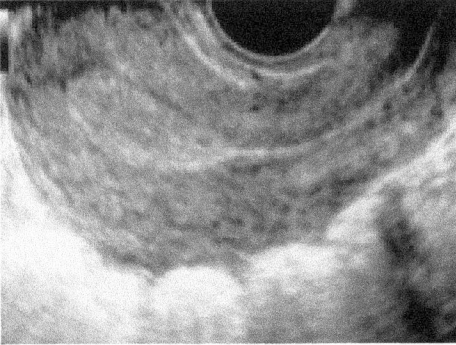 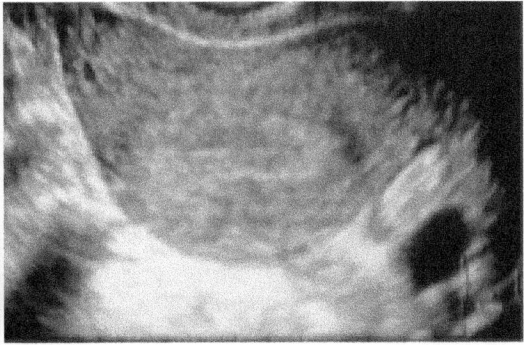

2.7a   **2.7b**

The above scans show a thickened endometrium which can be seen before any IUGS.

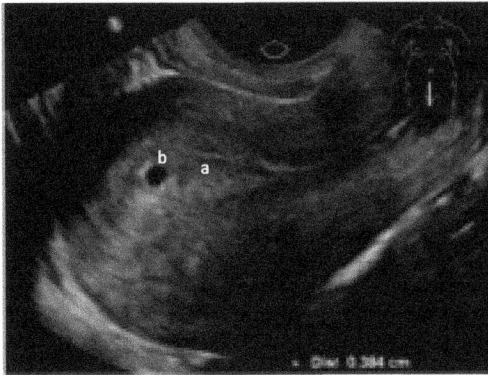 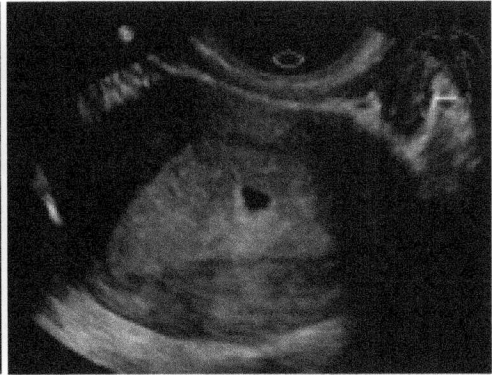

2.7c   **2.7d**

Then a tiny cystic entity appears in the endometrium as above (b in 2.7c - d).

a-thickened endometrium, b- possible gestational sac

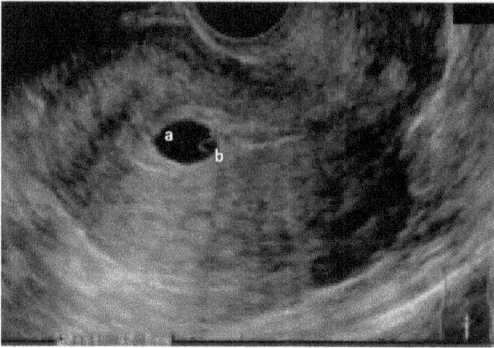 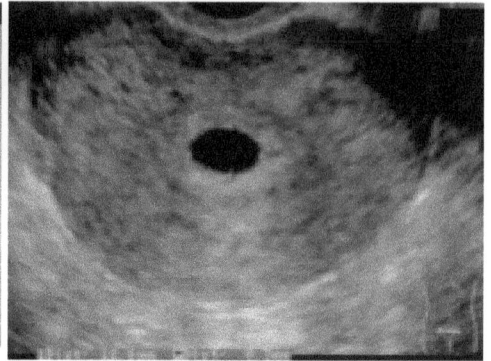

2.7e   **2.7f**

Then a bigger IUGS and tiny YS appear. *a- intrauterine gestational sac, b- yolk sac*

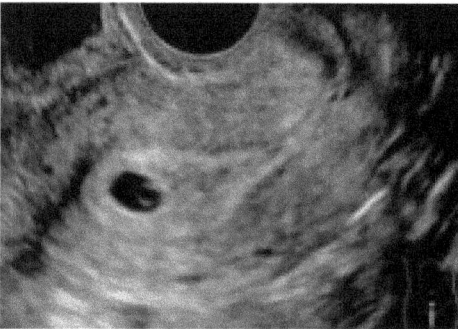 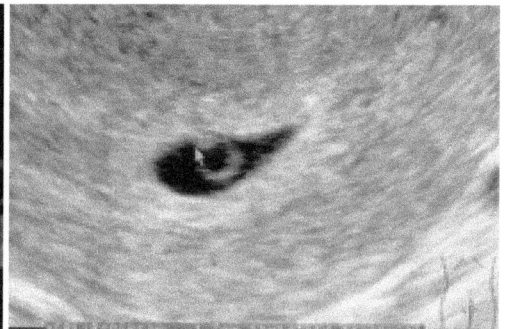

2.7g   **2.7h**

Five weeks and five days' gestation (5+5/40). Note the arrow pointing to the tiny embryonic pole (EMP). (This is the 'diamond ring' sign). EHB was also seen in this case.

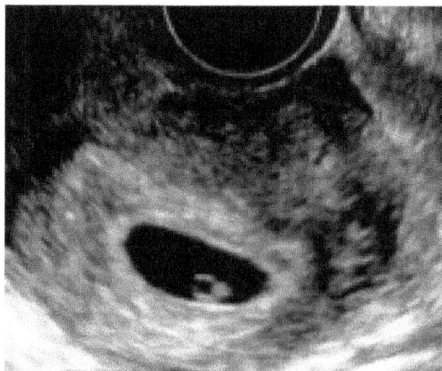

2.7i

GA = 6+/40. IUGS, YS and embryonic pole. This is the 'diamond ring' appearance.

Yolk sac (YS)

The YS is seen on ultrasound from 5/40 until the end of the first trimester.

The upper limit for a normal YS diameter (between 5 and 10/40) has been quoted as 5.6mm.

The YS is seen outside the amniotic membrane from 8+/40.

Between 4 and 5/40, the YS transfers nutrients to the embryo, whilst the uteroplacental circulation is being established. Blood circulation starts in the wall of the YS and continues until haemopoiesis starts in the liver at about 8/40 GA.

Primordial germ cells appear in the YS wall by 5/40 and these later migrate to the developing sex organs.

By 6/40, the dorsal part of the YS is incorporated in the embryo as the primary gut. Its endoderm forms the epithelium of the trachea, bronchi, lungs and gastrointestinal tract (GIT).

Ultrasound-reporting packages are available that can assign/estimate GA using the YS measurement.

7+/40

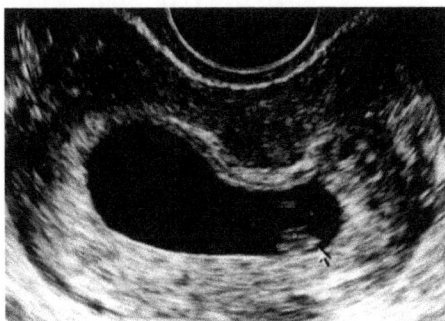

2.7j *GA =7/40. CRL =8.8mm. EHB seen.*

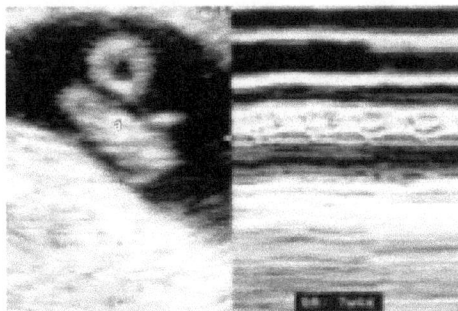

2.7k

Embryonic heart is seen as three echogenic parallel lines in the embryonic thorax at this stage. *a- heart*

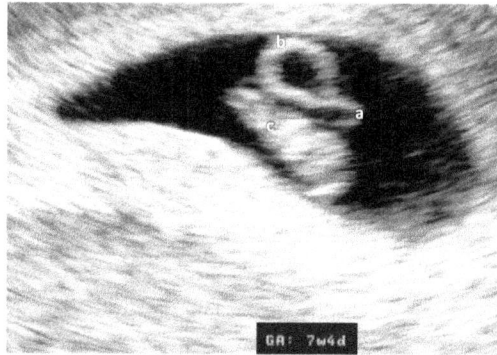

2.71

Note the vitelline duct which connects the embryo to the YS at this GA (7+4 in the above image). *a-vitelline duct, b-yolk sac, c-embryo*

Vitelline duct

- The vitelline duct is also called the yolk stalk or omphalomesenteric duct
- It connects the primitive gut to the YS
- The paired vitelline arteries and veins accompany the vitelline duct to provide blood supply to the YS

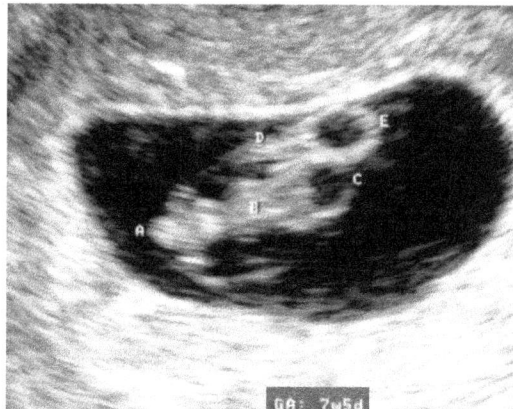

2.7m

A – rump. B – heart. C – crown. D – vitelline duct. E – yolk sac.

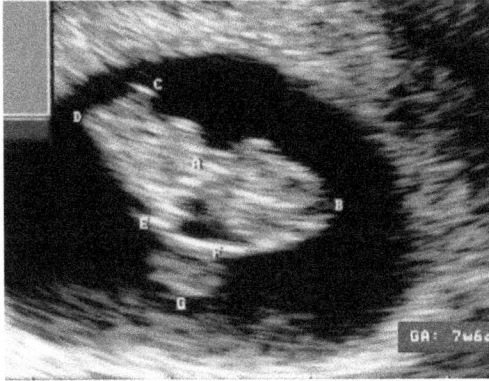

2.7n

A – heart. B – crown, C – lower limb bud, D – rump, E – upper limb bub,
F – amniotic membrane, G – yolk sac

8+/40

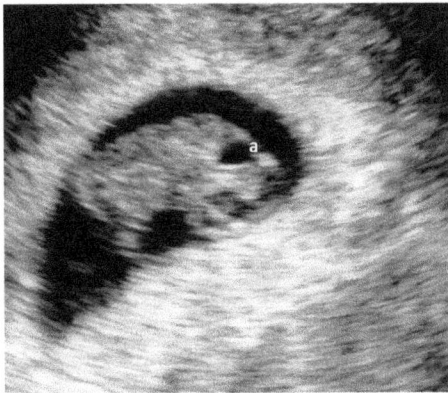

2.7o

GA = 8+2/40 – head showing a single cavity. a-rhombencephalon

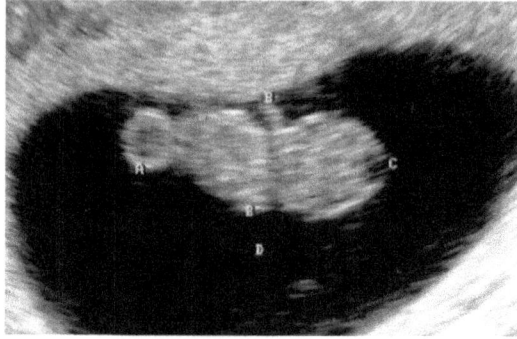

2.7p *GA by CRL = 8+3/40. A – yolk sa, B – primitive upper limb buds, C – crown, D - amniotic membrane*

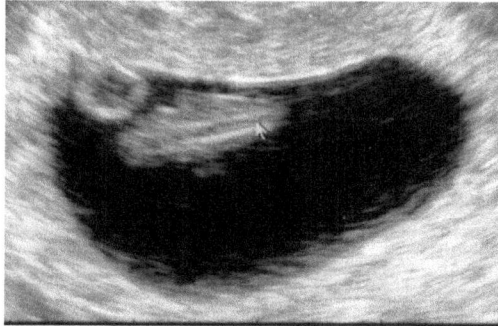

2.7q *8+3/40. Spinal canal*

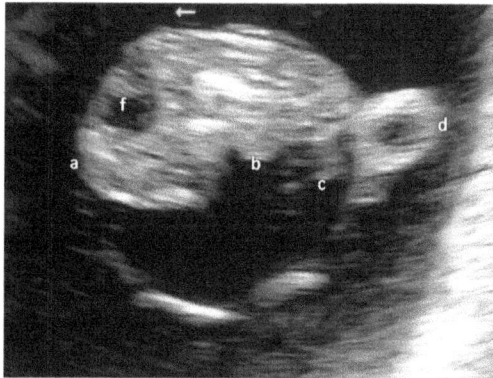

2.7r
CRL = 18.6mm = 8+4/40. *a-crown, b- primitive upper limb bud, c -lower limb bud, a- yolk sac, d- yolk sac, e-amniotic membrane, f-rhombencephalon.*

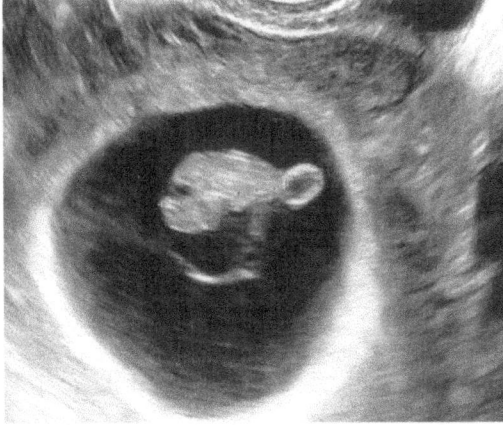

2.7s *Gestational sac, amniotic membrane, yolk sac @ 8+4/40*

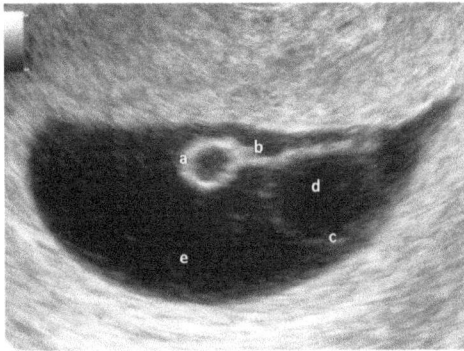

2.7t *8+4/40 – a-yolk sac, b- vitelline duct, c-amnion, d-amniotic cavity.*
e- chorionic cavity

8+5/40

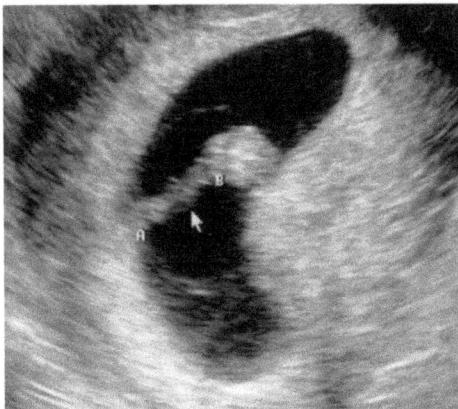

2.7u *8+ 5/40 A – cord insertion to placenta; B – cord insertion to the umbilicus.*

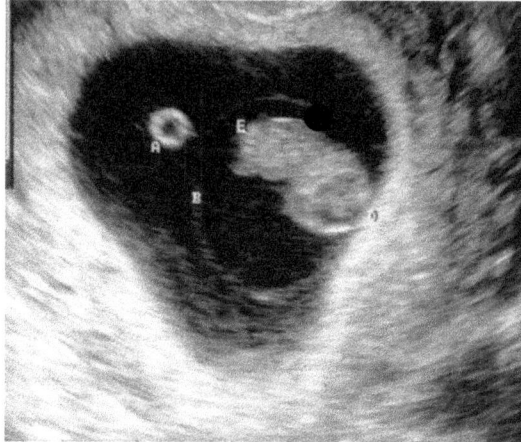

2.7v *A – yolk sac, B – amniotic membrane, D – crown, E – rump*

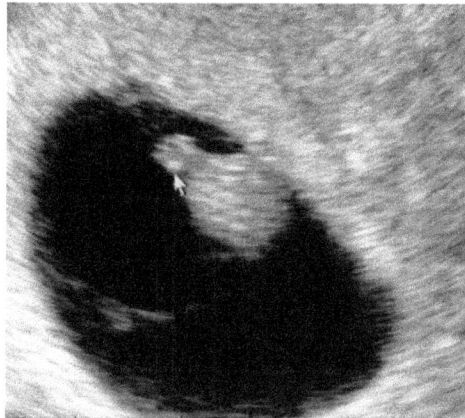

2.7w *TS abdomen showing physiological midgut herniation – a normal appearance for this stage of pregnancy*

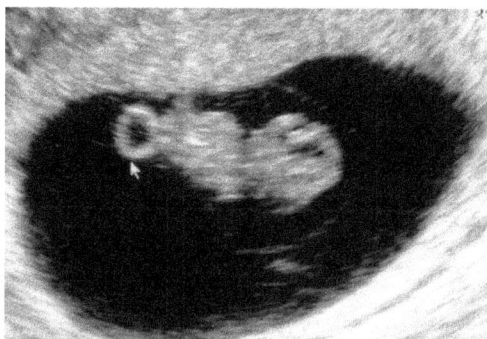

2.7x *Arrow pointing to the yolk sac*

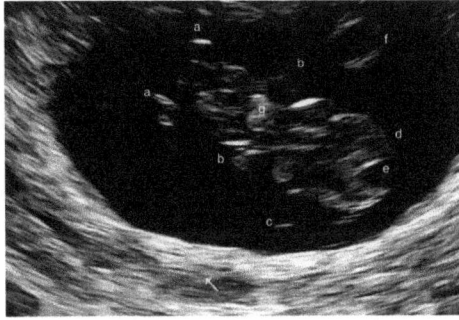

2.xb

***a**-lower limb bud, b-upper limb bud, c-amniotic membrane, d- amniotic fluid,
e- rhombencephalon. f- yolk sac, g- heart*

8+6/40

Spinal canal @ 8+6/40

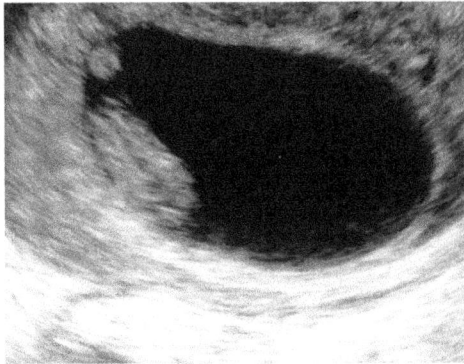

2.7y

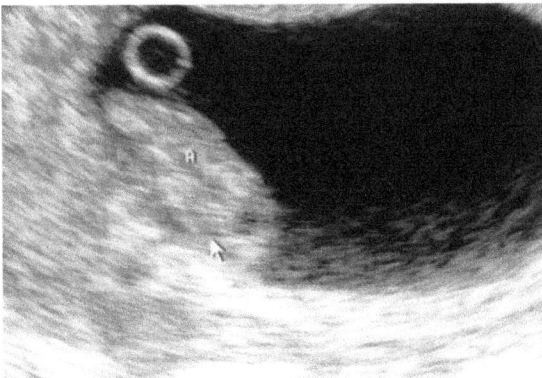

2.7z   *a-spinal canal.*

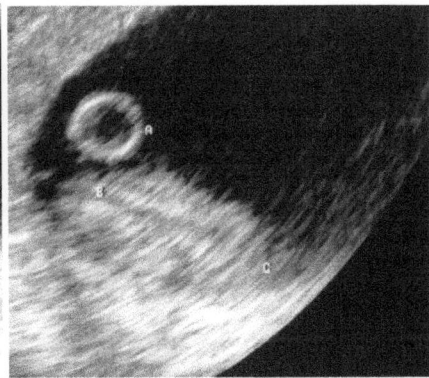

2.7za *a-yolk sac, b-spinal canal,
c-head*

9+/40

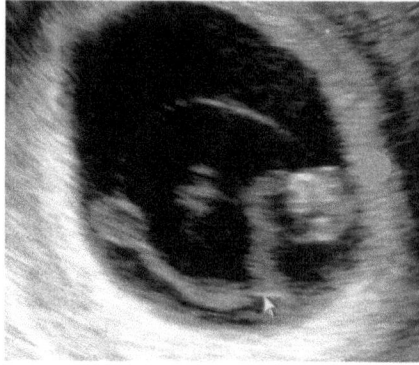

2.8a

9+1. Arrow pointing to the cord

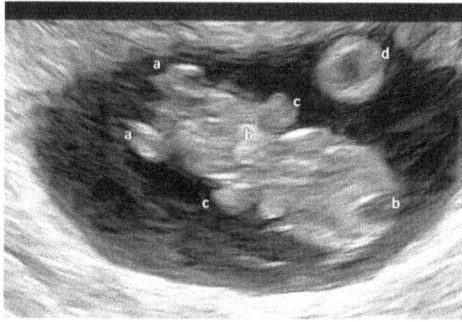

2.8b

a – lower limb bud, b – heart, c – upper limb bud, d-yolk sac.

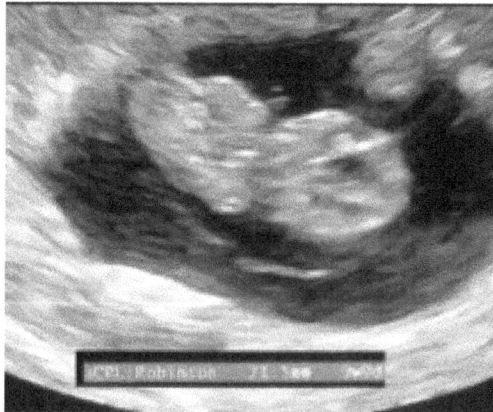

2.8c

GA by CRL = 9/40

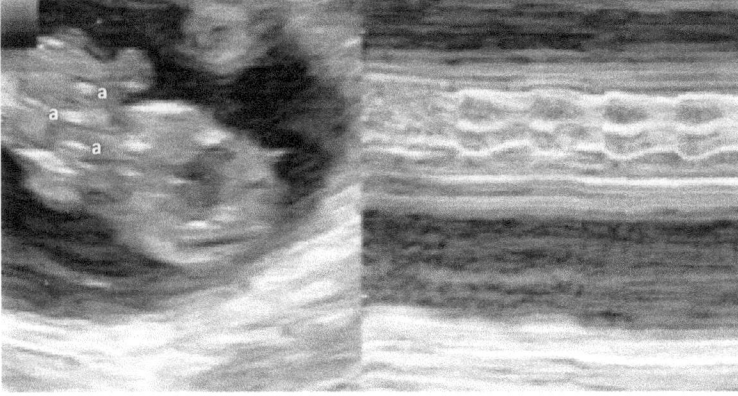

2.8d

Note the three parallel echogenic lines at the level of the heart – a above

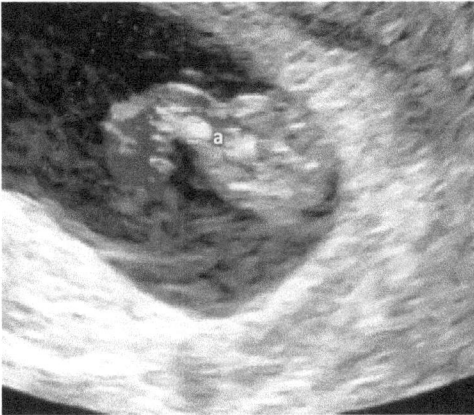
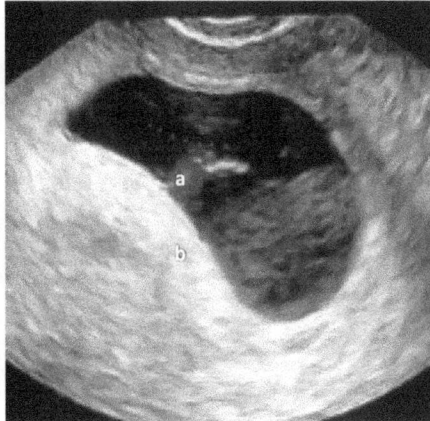

2.8e   **2.8f**

a - CI @ 9/40 to embryonic abdomen.

a-cord insertion to embryonic abdomen in 2.8e. a-cord insertion to the placenta, b-placenta 2.8f

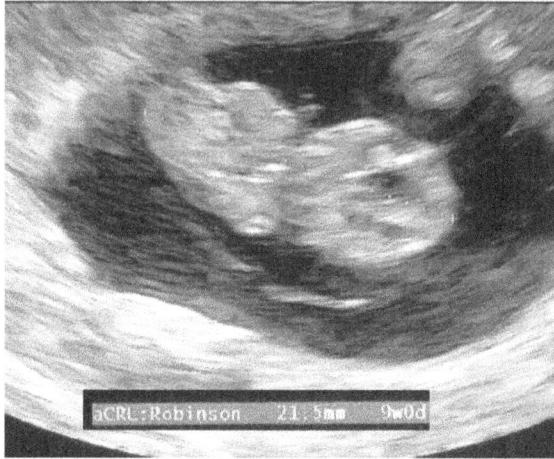

2.8g

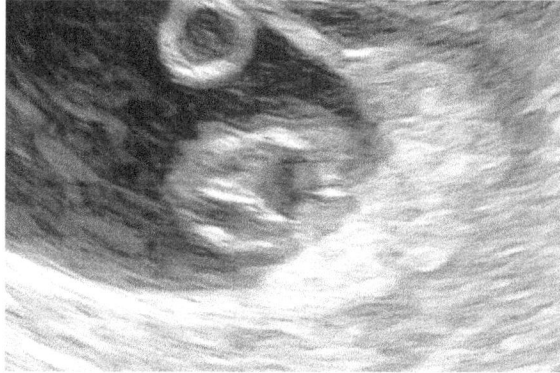

2.8

TS crown

10+/40

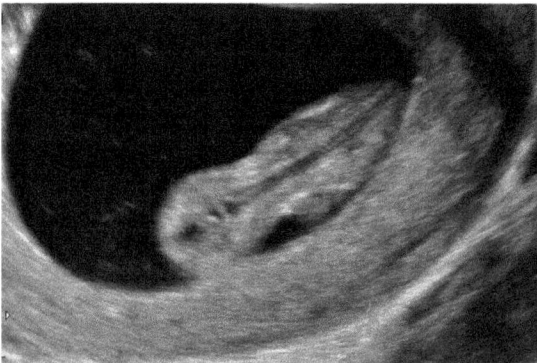

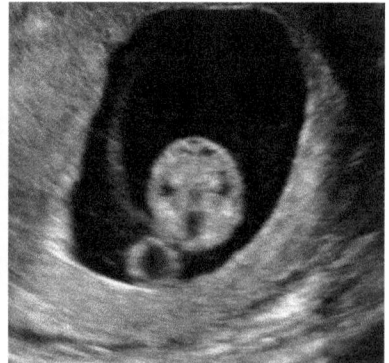

2.8i

Spinal canal @10+3/40.

2.8j

TS head @10+3/40.

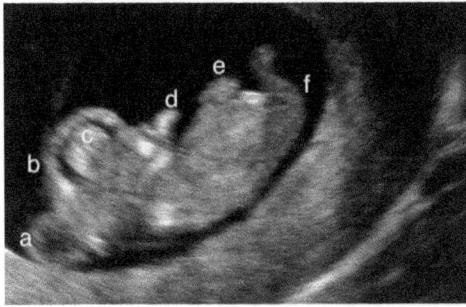

2.8k

sagittal view@10+3/40

a – yolk sac. b – cr own. c – choroid plexus. d – hand. e – gut. f – rump

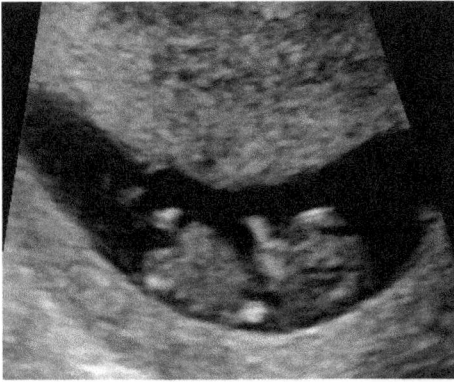

2.8l *10+3/40*

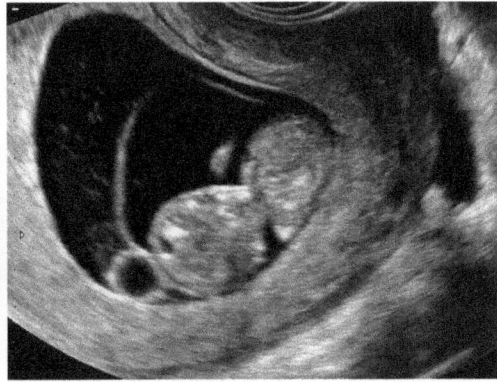

2.8m *10+3/40*

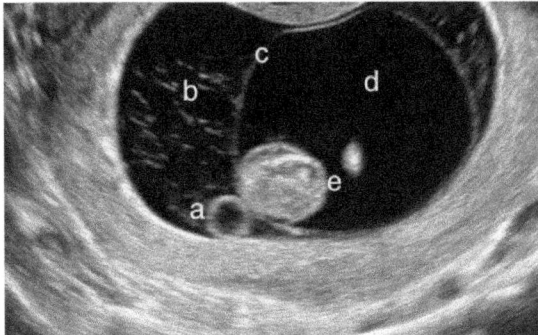

2.8n *10+3/40 a – yolk sac outside the amniotic membrane. b– amniotic fluid.*
c – amniotic membrane. d – chorionic fluid. e – fetal head.

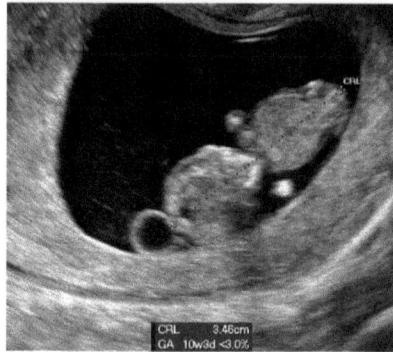

2.8o *GA = 10 +3/40*

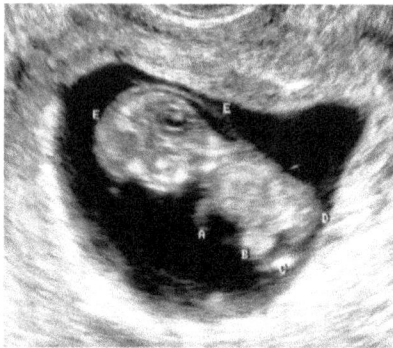

2.8p *GA = 10 +3/40*

A – upper limb bud. B – physiological midgut herniation. C – lower limb bud. D – rump. E – crown. F – skin covering at the neck.

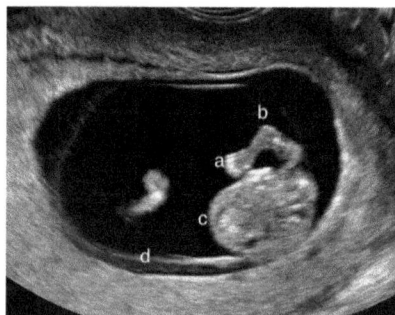

2.8q

a- Hand, b- elbow, c - amniotic membrane, d - head @ 10+ 3/40
Same fetus:

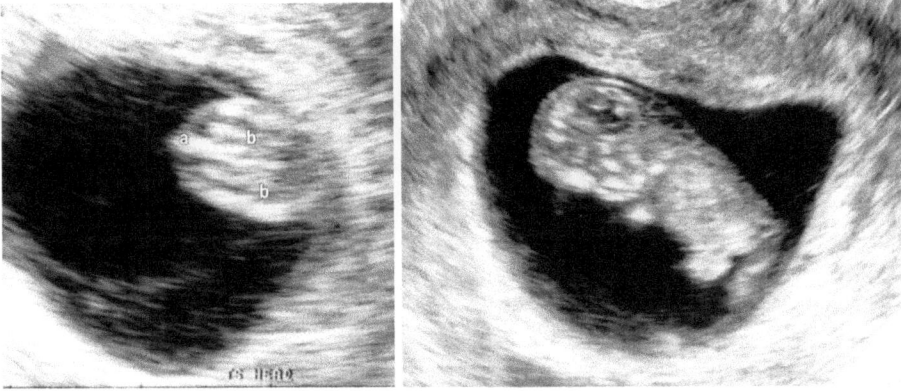

2.8r   **2.8s**

a-midline, b-choroid plexus

Amniotic fluid

- 99% of amniotic fluid is water
- It acts as a barrier to infection
- It allows symmetrical external growth of the fetus
- It prevents the amnion from adhering to the embryo
- It protects the embryo from injuries as any impacts from the mother are evenly distributed
- It protects the fetus from cord compression during fetal activity or uterine contractions
- It acts as a cushion to protect the fetus from the risk of limb and facial malformation
- It is composed of organic constituents such as protein, carbohydrates, fat enzymes, hormones, pigments, inorganic salts and fetal epithelial cells. In the later stages of pregnancy fetal meconium and urine are added
- It surrounds the fetus, allowing it to move freely which in turn encourages muscle development and limb movements

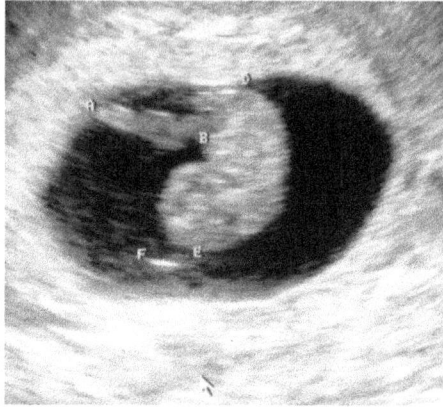

2.8t

A – cord insertion into the placenta. B – cord insertion into the umbilicus. D – rump.
E – crown. F – amniotic membrane.

11+ /40

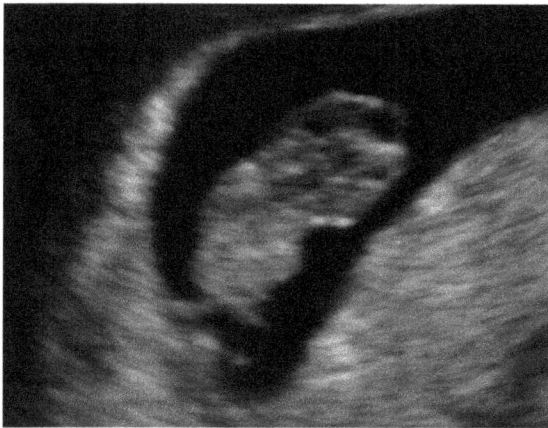
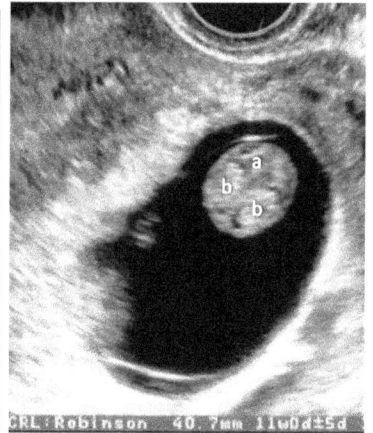

2.9a   **2.9b**

Fetal brain at 11/40
a-midline, b-choroid plexus

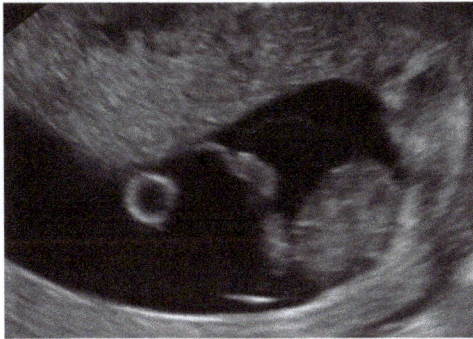

2.9c *Yolk sac, placenta, amniotic membrane*

12 +/40

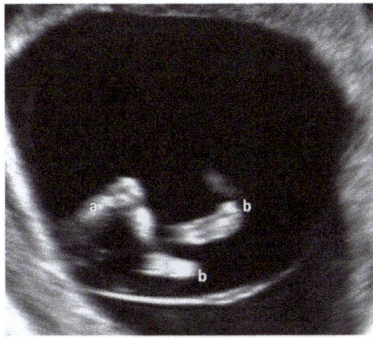

2.9d

Fetal leg and feet at 12+ 3/40. A-leg or femur, b-foot

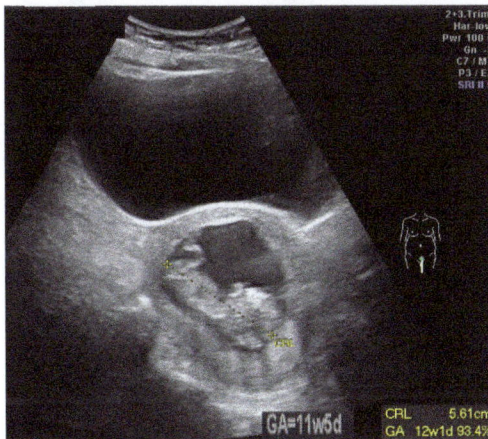

2.9e

TAS of an IUP in a retroverted uterus

Note the image resolution between a fetus in a retroverted uterus (2.9e) and another fetus in an anteverted uterus (2.9f). Both fetuses are similar in GA and both mothers had a full urinary bladder at the time of the examination.

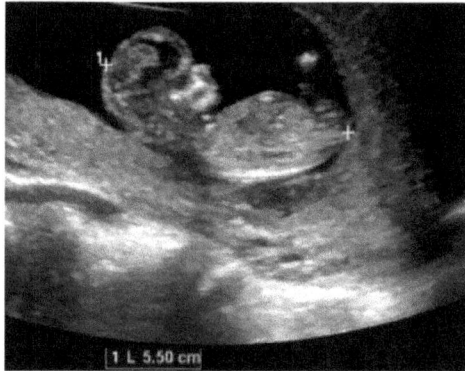

2.9f

TAS of an IUP in an anteverted uterus.

When a patient has a retroverted uterus, filling her urinary bladder actually pushes her uterus farther away from the TA probe; and, in order to obtain a good fetal assessment, a TV scan may become inevitable and performed with patient's consent.

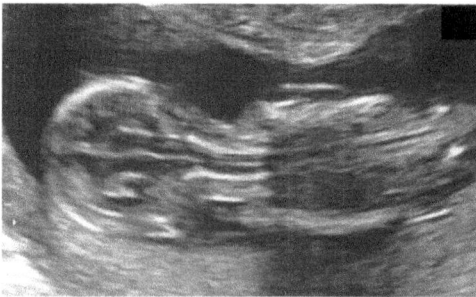

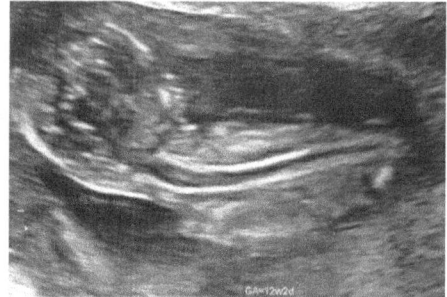

2.9h *12+4 /40*   **2.9g** *Spinal canal @ 12+2/40*

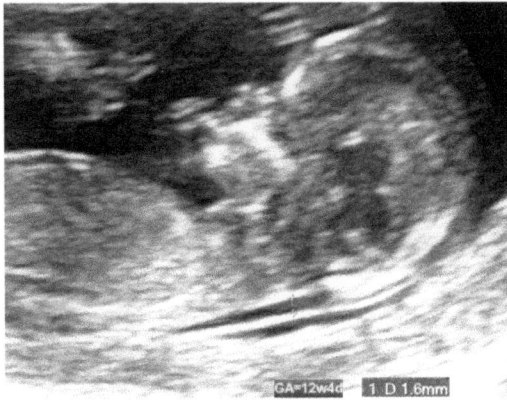

2.9i *Profile of the fetal face including the nasal bone.*

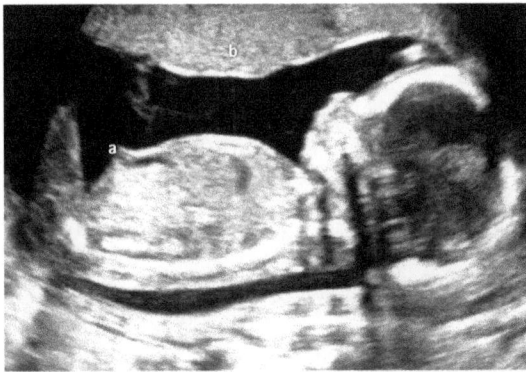

2.9j *Sagittal view of the fetus, showing the CI and anterior placenta.*
A-cord insertion, b-placenta

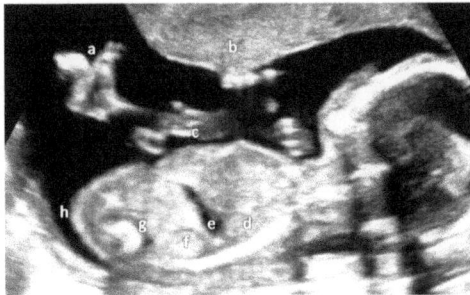

2.9k
Sagittal view of the fetus, showing a foot, cord, stomach, left kidney, left iliac crest,
left lung, anterior placenta and small intestine.
a-foot, b-anterior placenta, c-cord, d-left lung, e-stomach, f-left kidney, g-iliac crest,
h-rump/bottom

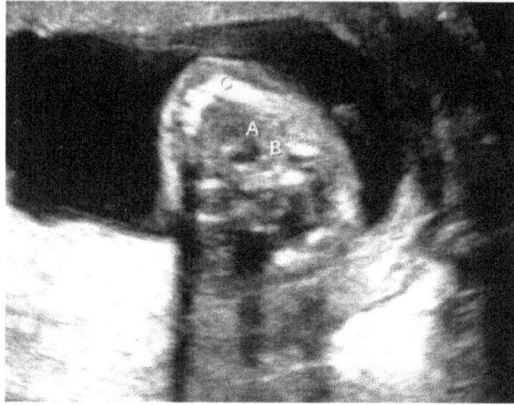

2.9l *A – soft palate. B – faucet. C – mandible.*

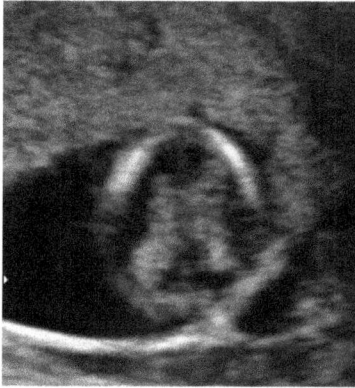

2.9m *Head at 12+5/40.*   **2.9n** *Head at 12+ 6/40.*

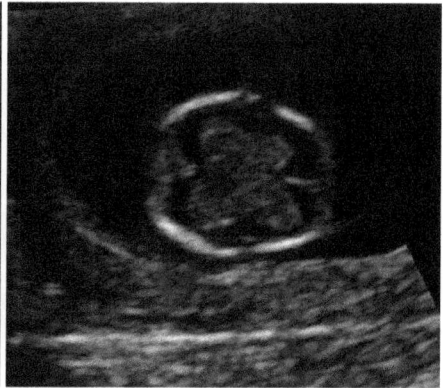

Different patients

Note the normal butterfly shape of the choroid plexus and the integrity of a normal skull outline.

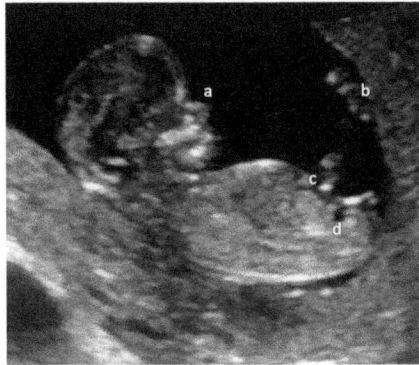

2.9o *a-facial profile, b-foot, c-cord insertion, d-urinary bladder*
12+4/40 – Note the urinary bladder, diaphragm, foot, cord insertion and facial profile.

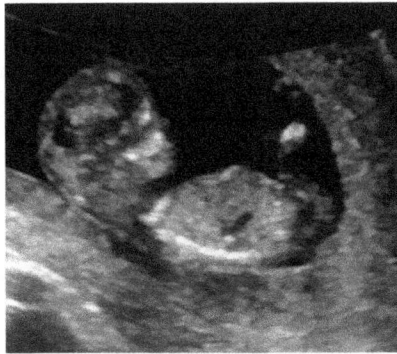

2.9p Note the fetal stomach at 12+4/40.

Documenting EHB or FHB and heart rates (bpm)

To confirm or otherwise show that the embryo or fetus is alive, the M-mode is used and a tracing is obtained at the level of the heart.

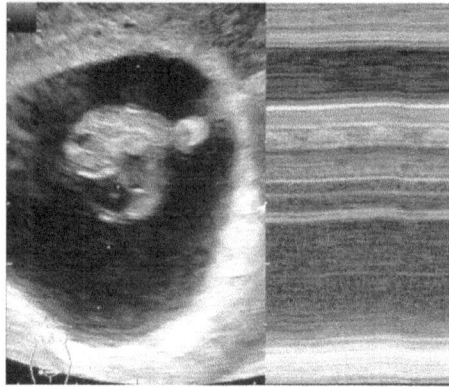

2.9q *M-mode to confirm that the embryo or fetus is alive*

Where the embryo or fetus is no longer alive straight Doppler lines are obtained.

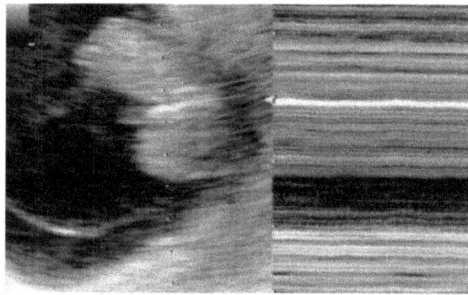

2.9r *M-mode demonstrating no FHB*

The embryonic or fetal heart beats (EHB or FHB) can be measured and the value obtained can be plotted on the appropriate EHR or FHR graph. This might become necessary especially where there is a suspicion of slow or too fast EMR or FHR.

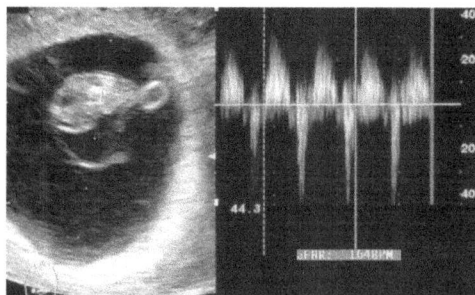

2.9s

EHR or FHR acquisition

It is believed that the peak mean heart rate of 175 beats per minute (bpm) occurs at 9 weeks' gestation, and thereafter decreases to 166 bpm at 12 weeks.

Bradycardia

It is believed that the embryo has bradycardia when:

At CRL < 5mm if the heart rate is < 80 bpm

At CRL 5–9mm if the heart rate is < 100 bpm

At CRL 10–15mm if the heart rate is < 110 bpm

EHB rate < 85bpm at 5–8/40

In order to avoid missing any gross abnormality of the fetus from 8/40, the fetus should always be scanned in two planes, sagittal and transverse from the head to the toes.

- The maternal adnexa should be checked in the first trimester so as not to miss any mass or cysts
- Inconclusive ultrasound findings or reports should be interpreted clinically with the b-hCG results and a follow-up scan organised 7–10 days later (or earlier if an ectopic pregnancy is suspected)
- A nuchal thickness of 3mm (9–12/40) is considered to be indicative of an increased risk of the fetus having trisomy 21 (Down's syndrome) or another chromosome anomaly or heart problems

Which fetal body part can be seen on ultrasound and when?

GA/40	Ultrasound recognises normal fetal part/anatomy	Comments
4+3	Intrauterine gestational sac (IUGS[i]) (TVS[ii])	Seen first as a small hypoechoic area within the echogenic/luteal phase endometrium
4.5 – 5	IUGS (TVS). Double decidual sac sign	With a b-hCG 1000 IU/mL
5	IUGS (TAS[iii]	When the b-hCG is 1800 IU/mL

5.5 – 6	Yolk sac (YS[iv])	First part/object to be seen in the GS[v]. Looks like a small wedding ring. Seen outside the amniotic membrane from 8+/40. The upper limit for a normal YS diameter of between 5 and 10/40 has been quoted as 5.6mm. It disappears by the end of the first trimester
6 – 6.5	Embryo	
6 – 6.5	EHB[vi] Seen as pulsations initially	Can be seen earlier with TVS. Seen first before the embryo and next to the YS. By 7+/40 the heart is seen as three hyperechoic lines in the embryonic thorax
6–8	A prominent cystic structure in the posterior cranial fossa	This is the rhombencephalon. This must not be mistaken for Dandy-Walker syndrome. It will later form the fourth ventricle
7	Amniotic membrane	It is seen as a bigger ring within the amniotic fluid and in it is the embryo. YS is always outside of this bigger ring. It fuses with the chorion by the end of the first trimester and sometimes up to 16 weeks GA
8–9	Primitive limb buds	A pair of upper and lower limbs buds
9–10+	Physiological midgut herniation. Feet, hands, umbilical cord, spinal canal, choroid plexus. Embryonic/fetal movement is seen	This must not be mistaken for omphalocoele. The choroid plexus appears as a bilateral echogenic structure in the fetal brain

11–13	Diaphragm, stomach, head with choroid plexus, midline and skull outline, urinary bladder, upper and lower limbs, five fingers, cord insertion, placenta, stomach, small intestine, heart (not in great detail), abdominal wall	

[i] intrauterine gestational sac; [ii] trans-vaginal scan; [iii] trans-abdominal scan; [iv] yolk sac; [v] gestational sac; [vi] embryonic heart beat.

Chapter Conclusion

It is important the sonographer has a good knowledge of anatomy and embryology because of the rapid growth and changes in ultrasound appearances especially in the first trimester. Sonographers should also be proficient at performing both TAS and or TVS as the case may require.

Bibliography Chapter 2

Books

Lyons EA. & Levi CS. (2005) in Diagnostic Ultrasound. 3rd ed. Rumack CM, Wilson SR, Charboneau JW, Johnson JM. (editors). St. Louis, Missouri, USA, CV Mosby, Elsevier.

Peregrine E, Pandya P. (2005) in Diagnostic Ultrasound. 3rd ed. Rumack CM, Wilson SR, Charboneau JW, Johnson JM. (editors). St. Louis, Missouri, USA, CV Mosby, Elsevier.

Shepherd GW. (1995) in Ultrasonography: An Introduction to Normal Structure and Functional Anatomy. Curry RA & Tempkin BB. (editors). USA, Saunders Company.

Articles

Andrews H. (1993) Normal First Trimester Appearance using Transvaginal Ultrasound. BMUS Bulletin: 1(3):8–12.

Axiana C, Zoppi MA, Ibba RM, et al. (2007) 3–4D Ultrasound in the First Trimester of Pregnancy. Available at: Donald School Journal of ultrasound in Obstetrics and Gynaecology, July – Sept: 1 (3):1–7. http://www.jaypeejournals.com/eJournals

Baby Centre Medical Advisory Board. Abnormalities of the Uterus and Fertility. Available at: http://www.babycentre.co.uk/a1038163/abnormalities-of-the-uterus-and-fertility

Canzone G. Parlato M, Triolo L. (2007) 2D–3D Ultrasound in the Diagnosis of Uterine Malformations. Available at: Donald School Journal of Ultrasound in Obstetrics and Gynaecology, July – Sept: 1 (3):77–79. http://www.jaypeejournals.com/eJournals

Centini G, Rosignoli L, Faldini E, et al. (2007) Fetal Anatomy by 3–4D Ultrasound. Available at: Donald School Journal of Ultrasound in Obstetrics and Gynaecology, July – Sept: 1 (3):8–16. http://www.jaypeejournals.com/eJournals

Clinical Standards Committee. ISUOG Practice Guidelines: Performance of First-Trimester Fetal Ultrasound Scan. Available at: http://www.isuog.org/nr/rdonlyres/9225e408-c904–4a7f-84ae-812e456fbddd/0/isuog1sttguidelines2013.pdf

Goel A and Weerakkody Y, et al. Chorioamniotic Separation. Available at: http://radiopaedia.org/articles/chorioamniotic-separation

Luijkx T, Gaillard F. Uterus Didelphys. Available at: http://radiopaedia.org/articles/uterus-didelphys

Medical Disability Advisor- Paraovarian Cyst. Available at: http://www.mdguidelines.com/ paraovarian-cyst

Chapter 3
Early pregnancy ultrasound examination

In this chapter we shall be considering the following

- The Sonographer and communicating 'bad news'
- Calculating the GA using the LMP
- Indications for Emergency Ultrasound in Early Pregnancy
- Maternal cysts in pregnancy - what does it mean

The sonographer and communicating 'bad news'

Pregnancy, though not a disease, is a complicated process with many stages – in the early stages of pregnancy things may go wrong. It is important that the sonographer is able to identify and deal with such ultrasound identifiable problems that may occur in the early stages of pregnancy.

Dealing with obstetrics 'bad news' entails close teamwork, but sonographers are often to the fore of such situations and have to make the diagnosis or convey the suspicion of expected or unexpected 'bad news'. Good communication skills to deliver such news to the patient or couple and being able to answer questions pertaining to the ultrasound examination or findings are essential. In some units, the sonographer is allowed single-handedly to give the bad news, whereas in other units another sonographer or an obstetrician must be called into the ultrasound room to confirm or refute the ultrasound findings. The sonographer is encouraged to work within the departmental protocols for communicating bad news.

Communicating bad news is a challenge that sonographers working in EPAGU have to deal with frequently in the course of their daily duties.
In obstetrics, there are two types of bad news both of which the sonographer may have to reveal to patients.

'Social bad news' is that which may bring unexpected trauma to the patient as a result of her current personal circumstances, e.g. multiple pregnancy or an unplanned pregnancy.

'Clinical bad news' may be because of the confirmation of anticipated findings, such as maternal instinct or suspicion of miscarriage, or unexpected findings during a routine scan, e.g. a missed abortion or miscarriage or and fetal abnormality.

It is important that the sonographer uses the word baby rather than embryo or fetus when talking to the patient. Early intrauterine death should be regarded as of equal significance to fetal death occurring at a later stage of pregnancy. There is no standard way of giving obstetric bad news or making the bad news good, but the bad news should be given gently, caringly and not abruptly. The patient should be given the opportunity of seeing the pregnancy condition on the television screen or monitor, as it is easier to explain to her what is wrong with her pregnancy and it affords her the opportunity to come to terms with the condition. Her questions relating to the ultrasound findings should be answered appropriately and when in doubt or not sure, the sonographer should politely encourage her to reserve the questions for the doctor in the unit.

A hardcopy of the ultrasound image should be offered to the patient. In some instances the patient may decline this offer. The patient's wishes are to be respected. Where the patient accepts the offer, a hardcopy of the pregnancy image should be given to the patient in a sealed envelope in case she may need it later. If she refuses the hardcopy, then it should be filed safely in her hospital notes.

Sonographers are human beings and can experience stress as a result of having to diagnose clinical bad news often under stressful conditions; these incidents, which can test one's abilities, may occur in succession in the EPAGU. To mitigate the effect of breaking bad news to a patient or couple, the sonographer can apply any or some of the following suggestions (not in any particular order):

- Finding out before or at the beginning of each scan all the relevant history for that particular pregnancy or patient
- Being prepared for the possibility of a poor outcome before each examination even when the scan is routine or a follow-up
- Being up to date with issues relating to professional practice
- Attending useful and relevant ultrasound counselling courses if need be
- Availability of written protocols
- It is good practice to have departmental policies on the confirmation of missed abortion or intrauterine death. For instance, should such events be left to the scanning sonographer or must he or she call another colleague to agree with the findings?
- Sharing stressful events with colleagues may make situations easier to tolerate
- Having more experienced colleagues at hand should there be need for a second opinion. This should not be seen as a weakness, but as strength and credibility as some ultrasound findings are uncommon and not straightforward
- Good teamwork with the clinicians and midwives is essential
- Having regular audit or multidisciplinary meetings in the unit and

discussions on the outcomes of abnormal or suspicious findings
- Staying in good health
- Identifying and using personally designed stress management strategies
- Being able to access independent hospital network support if and when needed

Clinical indications for emergency ultrasound in pregnancy

Patients who attend an early pregnancy unit (EPU) do so because they may be unsure of their LMP; their pregnancies are of a 'high risk' category; or they have had a previous bad or current bad obstetric history or experience associated with any of the following conditions:

- ? Ectopic pregnancy
- ? Molar pregnancy
- Poor obstetric history
- Unknown or unsure LMP
- Previous molar pregnancy
- Previous ectopic pregnancy
- Following fertility treatment
- History of recurrent miscarriage
- IUCD and +ve pregnancy test result
- Pregnancy of unknown location (PUL)
- Following assault or domestic violence
- Following accidents including 'bad falls'
- Patients with known severe haemophilia
- Nausea ± vomiting, hyperemesis gravidarum
- Maternal anxiety, e.g. previous missed abortion/miscarriage
- Abnormal vaginal bleeding and positive pregnancy test result
- Abdominal pains ± vaginal bleeding until 18 weeks gestation
- Generalised or local pelvic pains with +ve pregnancy test result

Patients who attend for emergency scans often have a high level of anxiety about what is happening with their pregnancy. Their emotions and hormone levels may be running high. The aims of scanning these patients are as follows
- Confirm pregnancy or otherwise
- Confirm the pregnancy location

- Confirm how many heartbeats,embryos or fetuses are present
- Date the pregnancy
- Assess the adnexa
- Assess any cause for pain or bleeding
- Assess any pregnancy complications
- Provide any seen ultrasound answer to the examination request
- Diagnose any obvious ultrasound recognisable embryonic or fetal abnormality appropriate for GA
- Assess the effect of assaults, accidents or 'bad falls' on the pregnancy
- Reassure the patient or couple where possible
- Suggest any follow-up scan that may be necessary

Ultrasound plays an important role in the diagnosis and management of these pregnancies.

Good communication with patients and their husbands or partners is an essential skill that sonographers should exercise in the course of their work. Talking to patients will relieve anxiety and make them more relaxed and cooperative. Conversation also helps to obtain from the patient any relevant information that may be needed to interpret the ultrasound findings and reassure the patient of the sonographer's commitment to help her.

Sonographers should know how to perform the ultrasound examination to the highest professional standard; they should show tolerance and understanding when patients are distressed and they should be able to empathise with them. Performing scans can be challenging for the sonographer where the ultrasound findings are inconclusive and the patient or family puts pressure on a sonographer for a diagnosis or prognosis; or when the Sonographer does not feel adequate to communicate the ultrasound findings or established earlier in the scan any relevant obstetric history before starting the examination

Calculating GA using the LMP

Before commencing the ultrasound examination, sonographers should introduce themselves to the patient or couple, check the patient's details and the reason for the scan (if known); they should also briefly explain the procedure to the patient and obtain the relevant consent for the scan.

The patient should be asked certain questions including: the date of her LMP if she knows it, the regularity of her menstrual cycle, if she was on the contraceptive pill or a contraceptive injection within 3 months prior to the pregnancy, was the pregnancy conceived naturally or otherwise, and any other relevant history that may affect the examination. The departmental protocol regarding 'chaperoning for TV scans' is to be adhered to at all times.

The LMP should not be used to calculate GA, especially when the monthly period prior to the pregnancy is unknown, the menstrual cycle is irregular, unsure; if the patient conceived less than 3 months from coming off the pill, whilst she was breastfeeding, with an IUCD in situ, or after a recent miscarriage or if she conceived with fertility treatment.

The LMPs cannot be used when a patient has conceived by IVF or ICSI infertility treatments. This is because there are many protocols for achieving the pregnancy, such as short, long, day 1, day 21. It is better to ask the patient her given EDD as often the fertility team would have already given her this information. When the EDD has not been established, then the patient should be asked when the embryo transfer took place and at what days post-fertilisation it was done. This information should be documented and used to calculate the EDD.

Let us consider how the same LMP may not give the same EDD in the following patients. Patients A – E have the same LMP which is 23/10/2017. You have been asked to calculate their GA on 10/01/2018.
1. Patient A has a normal 28-day cycle
2. Patient B has three to four periods per year
3. Patient C has a 35–42-day cycle
4. Patient D conceived by IVF
5. Patient E has a 21-day cycle
Please calculate the GA for each patient prior to her scan today (10/01/2018).

It is important that the GA of a pregnancy be established prior to the scan so that the ultrasound findings can be correlated to or with the calculated GA.

Answers

1. Patient A has a normal 28 days cycle. GA – 11+3/40
2. Patient B has three to four periods per year – GA cannot be calculated, as her ovulation date cannot be predicted
3. Patient C has – 35–42-day cycle– 10+3/40 -9+3/40
4. Patient D conceived by IVF. GA will depend on the date of the embryo transfer and the age of the embryo on the day of transfer
5. Patient E has a 21-day cycle. = 12+3/40

GA and EDD are normally based on a predicted ovulation date, which is influenced by the length of the menstrual cycle. The reason for the differences in the EDD above is due to the predicted or assumed different ovuation date. In patients who conceive through IVF, because of the variety and length of the possible protocols used, the only certain date is when the embryo is transferred, which is similar to the ovulation date used in calculating the natural conception GA.

In this section we shall consider some of the reasons why patients are referred for a scan at EPAGU and present some examples:

Ectopic pregnancy

Ectopic pregnancy (EP) is a pregnancy that is implanted outside the fundus or body of the uterus. It accounts for approximately 1.15% of all pregnancies in the United Kingdom. Most ectopic pregnancies are tubal, but ectopic pregnancy can be cornual, ovarian, cervical, within a uterine scar, intraabdominal or heterotopic. Undiagnosed or missed ectopic pregnancy can cause maternal death. Finding an intrauterine pregnancy cannot exclude a co-existing heterotopic pregnancy, especially in patients who conceive with fertility treatment and who have more than one embryo transferred. The quoted rate is 1 in 100 compared to 1 in *3800/3200 in patients who conceive naturally. Other patients who are prone to ectopic pregnancy include those who:

- Are smokers
- Have had tubal or pelvic surgery
- Have tubal problems or tubal ligation
- Had infertility treatment or assisted conception
- Have endometriosis which may cause tubular damage

- Use emergency contraception in their current pregnancy
- Have previous pelvic inflammatory disease (PID) secondary to *Chlamydia trachomatis* or other sexually transmitted infections
- Conceived with an IUCD in place. An IUCD is able to prevent pregnancy in the uterus but is less effective in preventing a pregnancy in the uterine tube
- Conceive whilst using the progesterone-only pill (mini pill) as it alters the motility of the tube
- Had a previous ectopic pregnancy – rate quoted is up to 1 in 5 of spontaneous pregnancy after an ectopic pregnancy

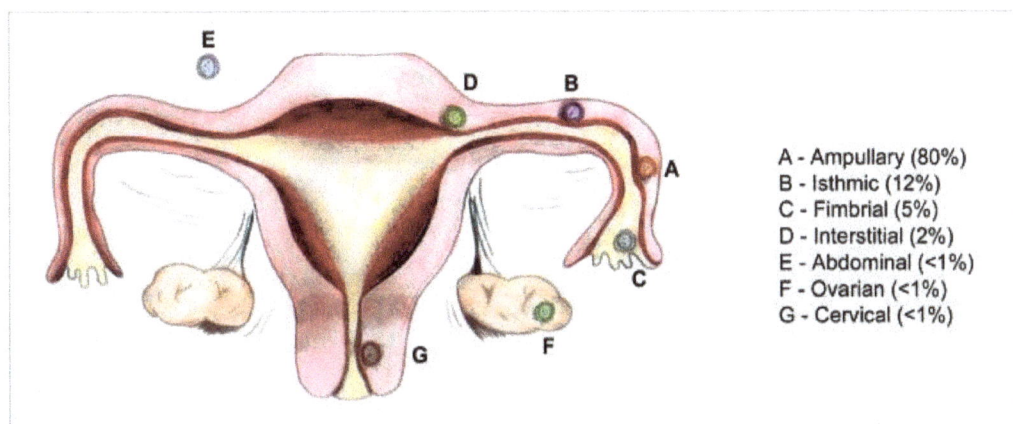

A - Ampullary (80%)
B - Isthmic (12%)
C - Fimbrial (5%)
D - Interstitial (2%)
E - Abdominal (<1%)
F - Ovarian (<1%)
G - Cervical (<1%)

Figure 3.1. Possible locations of ectopic pregnancies.
Used with the permission of the Ectopic Pregnancy Trust. (www.ectopic.org.uk)

Ultrasound signs of an ectopic pregnancy

- Empty uterus
- Tubal ring
- Adnexal mass
- Mass next to the ovary
- Complex fluid in the pelvis
- Decidual reaction in the endometrium
- Low-level echoed or free pelvic fluid
- Echogenic ring on the same side as the corpus luteum – not always
- Gestational sac, ± yolk sac with or without heartbeat outside the uterine fundus or body

* In a heterotopic pregnancy there will be an IUGS in the uterus but another ectopic pregnancy outside the uterus.

When the ultrasound findings are inconclusive, the β-hCG should be considered and used to interpret the ultrasound findings. Ideally when β-hCG levels exceed 1000 IU/mL a gestational sac (GS) should be seen using the TVS approach and with β-hCG of 1800 IU/mL a GS should be seen using the TAS approach. The β-hCG level doubles every 24–48 hours in a normal ongoing pregnancy.

With an ectopic pregnancy, the β-hCG may increase but at a lesser rate than expected. It may plateau or decline. The β-hCG level also declines following a spontaneous abortion that does not have uterine RPOC.

Any or all of the following factors may influence the detection of an ectopic pregnancy:

- Overlying bowel gas
- Shadows from fibroids
- Sonographer's experience
- Active bowels may be a challenge
- Patient's ability to tolerate a TV scan
- Quality or resolution of the images obtained
- Increased patient's BMI especially in early GA
- GA at the time of the scan. It may be easier to locate an ectopic later in pregnancy, e.g. at 8/40 than at 5/40

3.1. This patient was referred with a history of abdominal pains and light bleeding. She was known to have had previous c/sections. GA by LMP = 9+2/40.

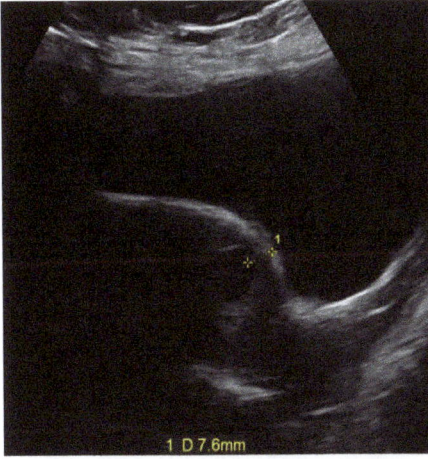

3.1a TAS

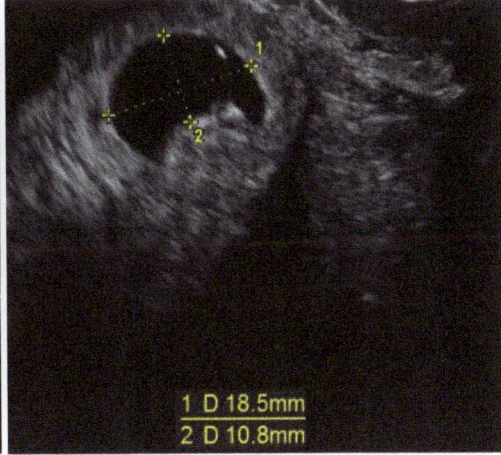

3.1b TVS

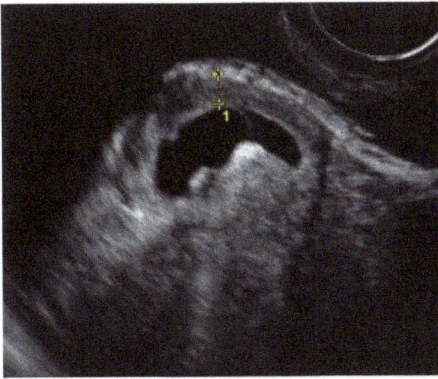

3.1c TVS

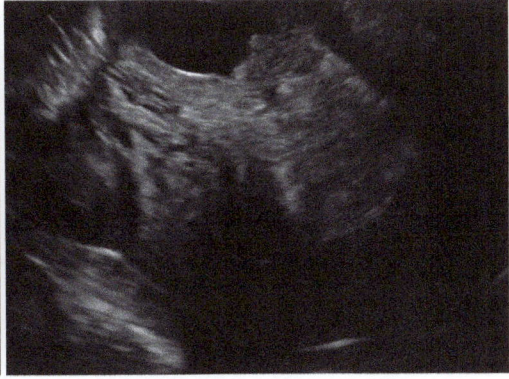

3.1d TVS

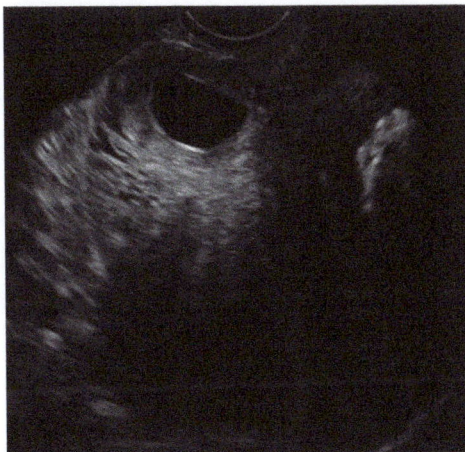

3.1e

Ultrasound findings: There is an IUGS located eccentrically in the anterior cervical area near where the expected previous caesarean section scar gestational sac is (3.1a–e). The IUGS measures approx. 19 × 11mm (3.1b–c). An approx. 8mm myometrial thickness is visualised in the anterior wall of the cervix (3.1a). There is little myometrium between the gestational sac and maternal urinary bladder. No obvious free fluid is demonstrated in the POD. The uterus appears heterogenous with a possible anterior or fundal fibroid – (3.1a, c, & e) measurements are not included.

Impression: Caesarean section scar pregnancy.
Differential diagnoses may include a cervical pregnancy or an ongoing abortion or miscarriage but this will be in the cervical canal not in the anterior cervical myometrium.
There is an intramural or fundal fibroid (measurements not included).

Caesarean section scar ectopic pregnancy
* Is rare, 1 in about 2000 pregnancies
* Rate might be increasing due to the rate of increasing caesarean sections
* Ultrasound findings of caesarean section scar ectopic pregnancy will demonstrate a gestation that is completely surrounded by both myometrium and fibrous tissue of the caesarean section scar and separated from the endometrial cavity and endocervical canal

3.2
This patient was referred for a dating scan. FHB and movements were seen but not shown here.

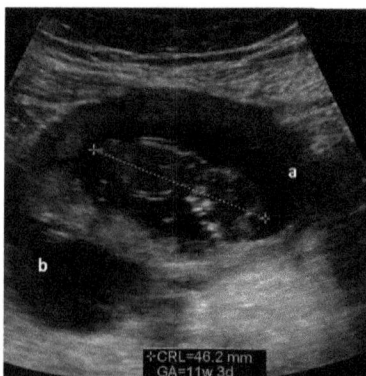

3.2a

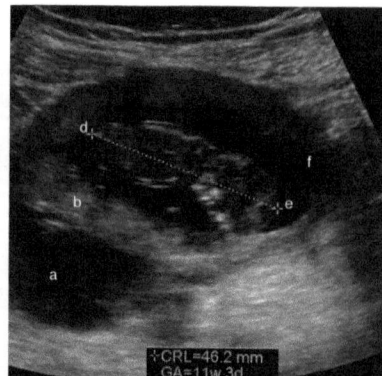

3.2b

3.2a a-thin myometrium, b- fluid collection. **3.3b** a - septated fluid, b - uterine myometrium, d - rump or bottom, e- crown or head, f- thin myeometrium

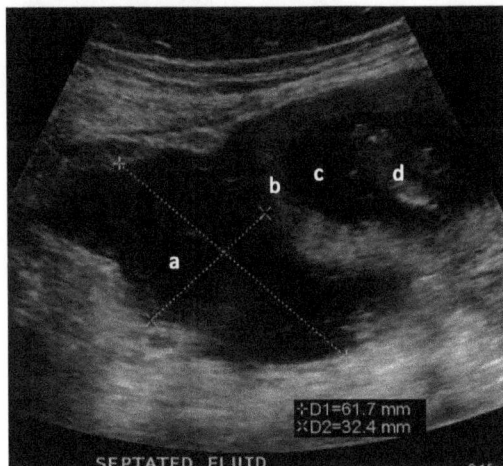

3.2c

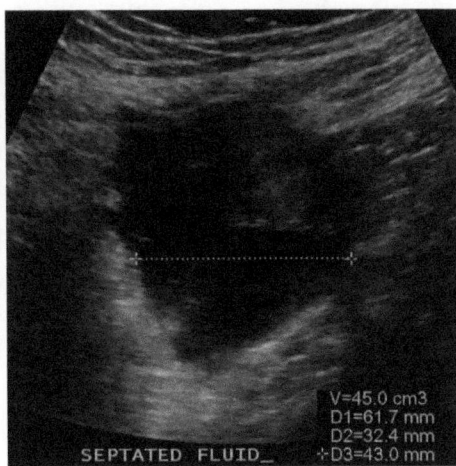

3.2d

a- irregular in outline septated fluid, b-shows some part of the gestational sac not completely surrounded by the myometrium c- gestational sac, d-embryo

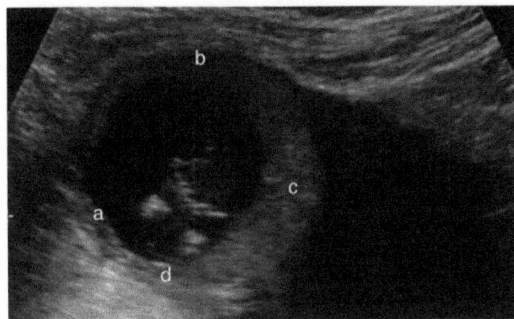

3.2e

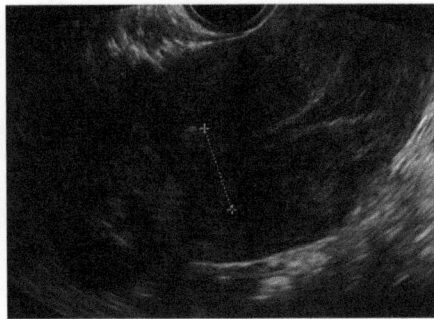

3.2f

Right adnexa a – no myometrium, b – thin myometrium, c – uterine myometrium d- thin myometrium

In 3.2f Endometrium ++ = 23mm

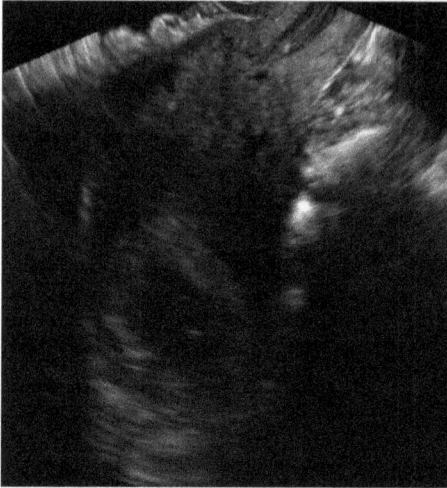

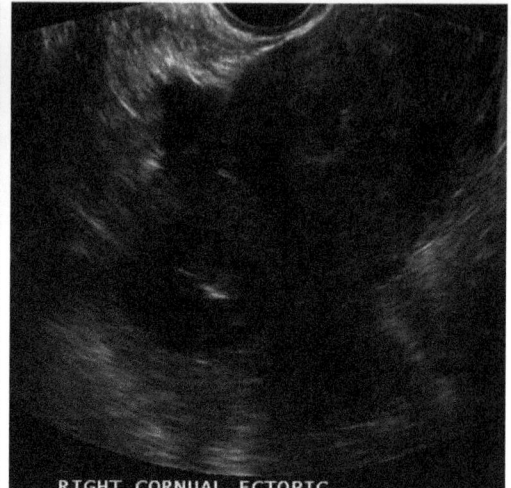

3.2g   **3.2h**

Ultrasound findings: The endometrium is 23mm thickened (3.2f) There is an eccentrically located gestational sac and fetal pole in the right adnexal with an incomplete or asymmetrical uterine myeometrium (3.2e-h) cornual / interstitial pregnancy seen (3.2g-h). CRL = 46.2mm = 11+3/40 (3.2a-b). Some multi septated fluid is seen around the GS measuring approx. 62 x 32 x 43mm (3.2c-d). This is suggestive of hemorrhage (3.2a -d).

Impression: Right cornual or interstitial pregnancy with some haemorrhage. Differential diagnosis will include – eccentric gestational sac and tubal ectopic pregnancy.

*This patient was asymptomatic at the time of her examination
* Right cornual or interstitial pregnancy was confirmed at surgery
Experts believe that:

- Intestitial or cornual pregnancy accounts for 2–4% of all ectopic pregnancies
- As the pregnancy lies within the interstitial portion of the Fallopian tube, it has the potential to grow larger than standard tubal ectopics by the time of presentation
- Cornual pregnancies are more prone to rupture in the second trimester of pregnancy
- There is a greater tendency of massive haemorrhage

- Maternal morbidity and mortality are higher due to late presentation and associated complications, especially haemorrhage
- Risk factors include previous intrauterine instrumentation

Ultrasound features of an interstitial or cornual pregnancy
- An eccentrically located gestational sac (GS) or an extrauterine gestational sac
- A GS surrounded by an incomplete or asymmetric uterine myometrium. Note a–c in 3k
- The endo-myometrial mantle or EMM (the distance from the outer part of the GS to the uterine wall) has been quoted as less than 5mm and in some quarters as less than 8mm
- Absence of a normally positioned intrauterine pregnancy
- A GS in the lateral portion of the uterus early in pregnancy and positioned above the fundus of the uterus in later pregnancy
- Heterogeneous mass in the cornual portion of the uterus
- 'Interstitial line' sign

3.3
Molar pregnancy

When a patient is sent for a scan in pregnancy with a clinical condition of nausea and vomiting or hyperemesis, one of the clinical conditions that needs to be confirmed or refuted is a molar pregnancy. Another is multiple pregnancy.

The ultrasound findings shown here are of a patient at 12+3/40. There was no history of vaginal bleeding in this pregnancy; both ovaries were not identified during the examination.

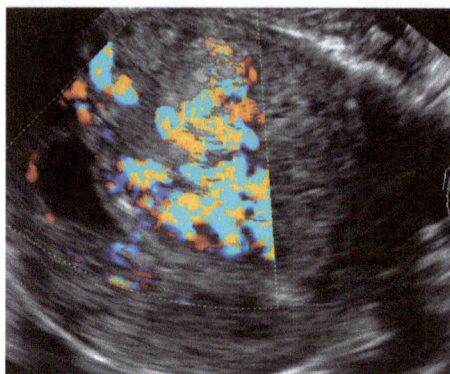

3.3a

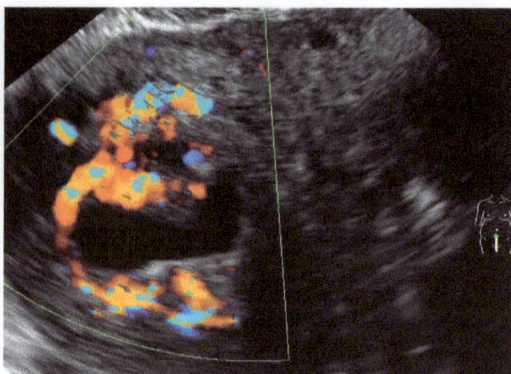

3.3b

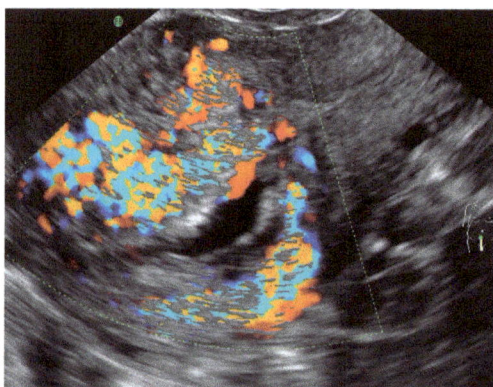

3.3c

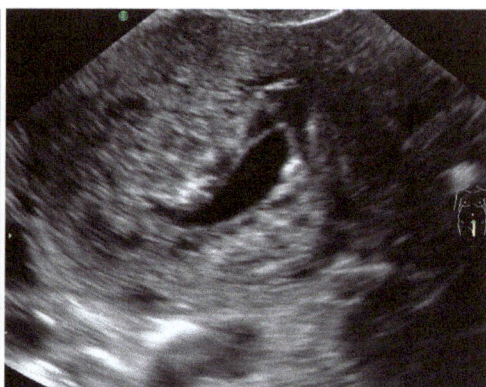

3.3d

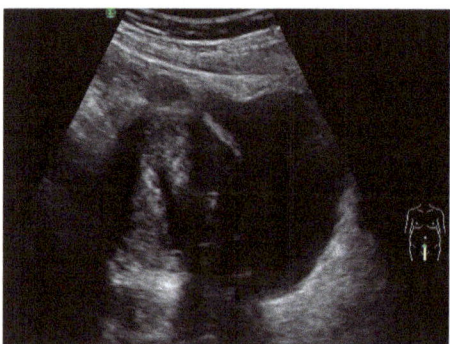

3.3e

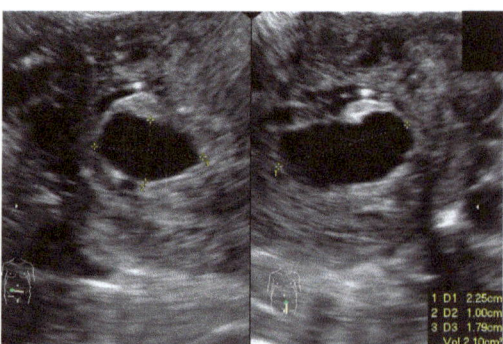

3.3f

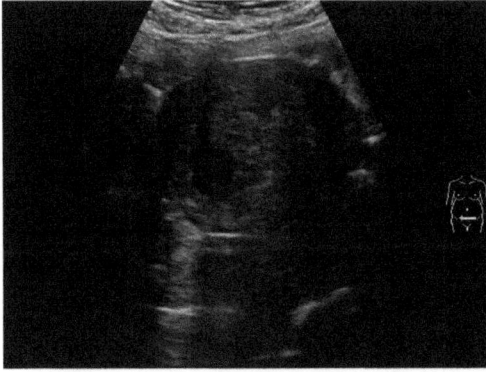

3.3g

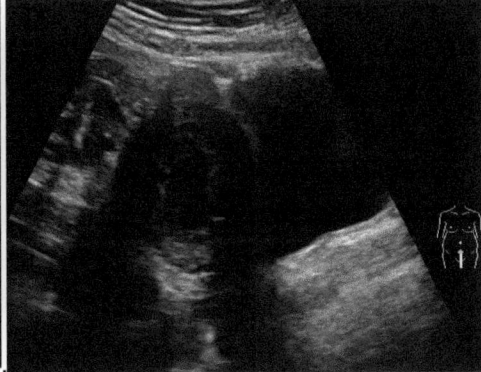

3.3h

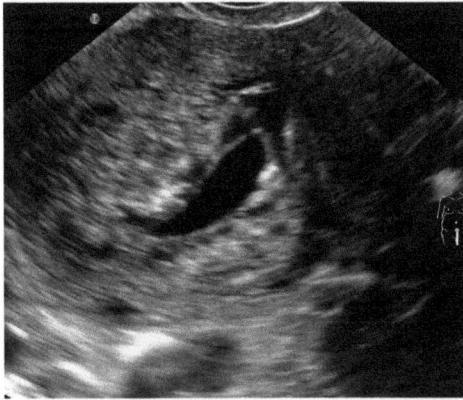

3.3i

Ultrasound findings: There is an elongated, slightly irregular in outline, small intrauterine cystic entity, ?IUGS. (3.3a–i). The volume of this ? IUGS = 2.10cm/mls (3.3f). Anterior to the ?GS is a predominantly vascular hyperechoic area that has some tiny cysts in it (3.3a–c, 3.3e, g, i). No obvious YS or EMP has been demonstrated.

Impression: Complete molar pregnancy. Differential diagnoses are – an anembryonic pregnancy or missed abortion or miscarriage.

- Follow-up laboratory histological tests did not show trophoblastic disease but missed abortion or miscarriage.

This patient's scan at 12+5 revealed these images (3.4a–e).

β-hCG levels was more than 90 000 IU/ mL at the time of the scan.

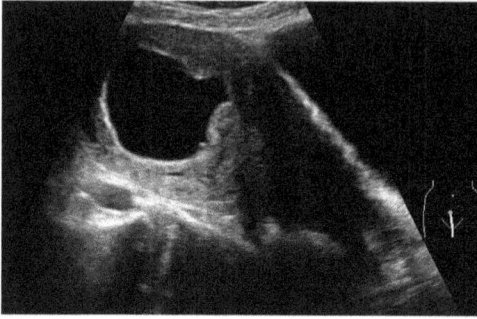

3.4a

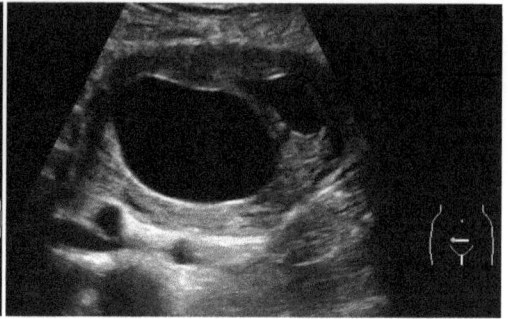

3.4b

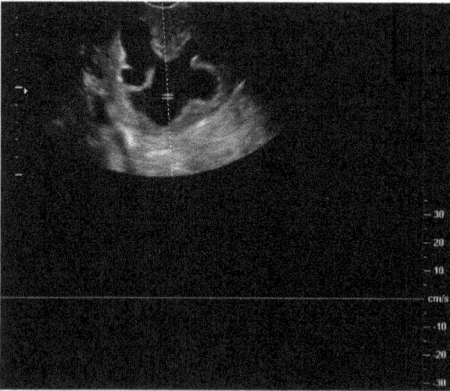

3.4c

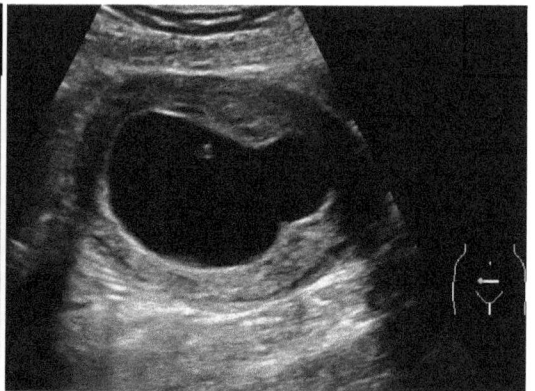

3.4d

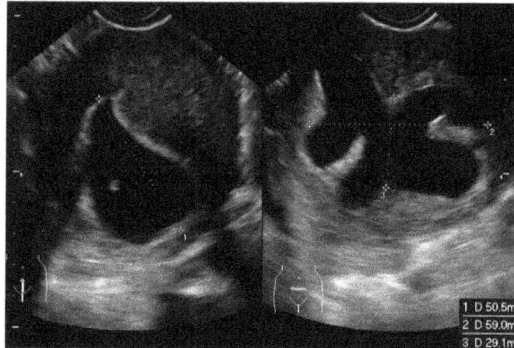

3.4e

Ultrasound findings: There is an irregular in outline gestational sac (3.4a–d) measuring approx. 51 × 59 × 29mm (3.4e). No yolk sac or embryonic pole is demonstrated.

Impression: ? molar pregnancy, ? anembryonic pregnancy.

* Histology confirmed that it was a partial molar pregnancy

A molar pregnancy occurs due to an abnormal fertilisation process

Patients who are more prone to a molar pregnancy include those who:

- Have had a previous molar pregnancy. For patients with one previous molar pregnancy the chance of another molar pregnancy has been quoted as 1 in 80 and in patients with two previous molar pregnancies the chance of another molar pregnancy is 1 in 6
- Are of increasing maternal age – over 50
- Very young females of reproductive age of Asian ancestry
- There is claim that it can be due to a nutritional deficit, such as a deficiency of protein, carotene or it may be caused by an ovulatory (ovulation) defect

Molar pregnancies can be

A complete mole: This is caused by a sperm fusing with an egg that has no DNA – genetic material. Such a fertilised egg will only grow the trophoblast – chorion. Usually there is no fetus, no placenta, no fluid and no amniotic membranes. The uterus is filled with the mole that resembles a bunch of grapes. The fluid-filled vesicles grow rapidly, which can make the uterus seem larger than it should be for gestational age. Vaginal bleeding can be seen and there is no placenta. Experts believe that advanced paternal age may be a risk factor for a complete molar pregnancy. A complete mole is entirely paternal in origin, with a karyotype of usually 46 XX.

- Patients with a complete molar pregnancy usually present with the typical symptoms of no periods, vaginal bleeding, hyperemesis, passage of grape-like vesicles per vagina and a uterus larger or smaller than dates.
- There may be pregnancy induced hypertension prior to 24 weeks or hyperthyroidism.

A partial molar pregnancy: Occurs when two sperms fertilise a normal egg. An embryo may or may not be seen. When the embryo is seen the placenta outgrows it. Experts claim that a partial mole predominantly has a triploid karyotype of 69XXX or 69 XXY or 69 XYY; however, a diploid karyotype may also exist.

It is possible to have a twin pregnancy with a normal fetus and a molar pregnancy. Rarely will the fetus survive.

With a partial molar pregnancy, patients are usually asymptomatic or may present with symptoms of a missed or incomplete abortion.

An invasive mole: This occurs where the trophoblast of a complete mole spreads outside the uterus. The patient is at risk of death from severe hemorrhage as the invasive molar villi may embolise to the lungs and brain.

Choriocarcinoma: This occurs where the trophoblast invades and spreads widely. Distant metastases are common in the lungs, liver, brain, kidneys, GIT and pelvic organs. It may follow a complete mole and rarely may follow a normal pregnancy, miscarriage or termination of pregnancy (TOP). It is a rare malignancy with a quoted incidence rate of 1 in 30 000 – 1 in 50 000 pregnancies.

The ovaries should be checked to confirm ovarian enlargement with theca lutein cysts, which are a common finding in about 40% of moles.

3.42 This patient was referred with a history of anxiety and pvb. Natural conception. GA by LMP = 5+4/40.

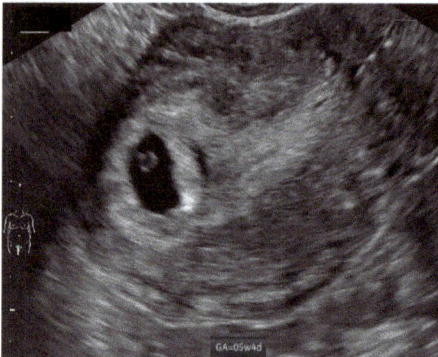

3.42a

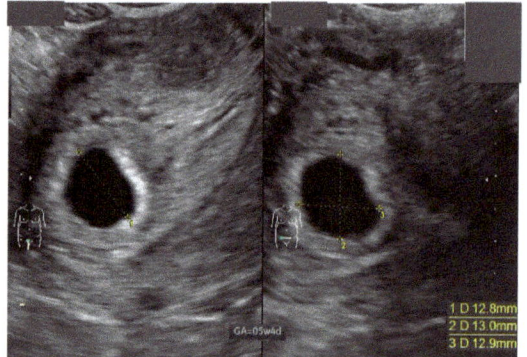

3.42b *(13 x 13 x 13mm)*

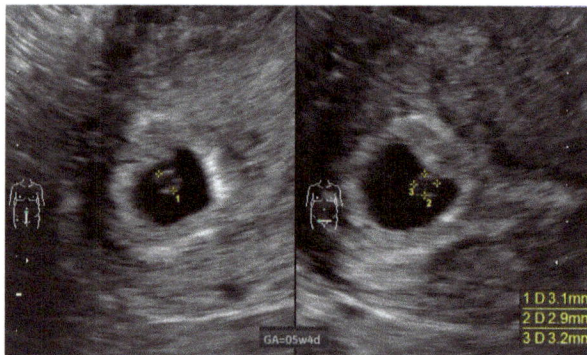

3.42c *(3 x 3 x 3mm)*

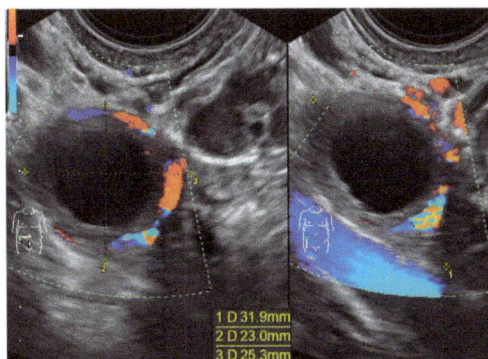

3.42d (32 x 23 x 25mm)

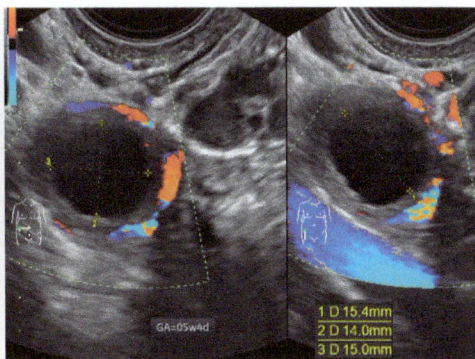

3.42e (15 x 14 x 15mm)

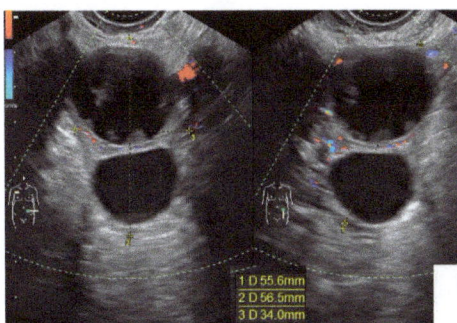

3.42f (56 x 56 x 34mm)

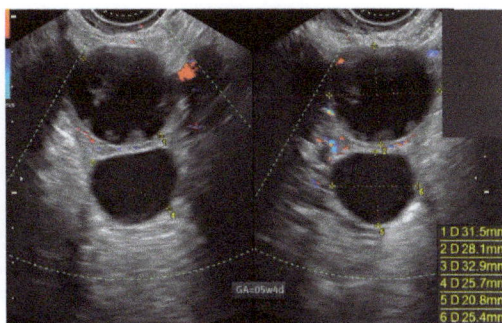

3.42g (32 x 28 x 33mm, 26 x 21 x 25mm)

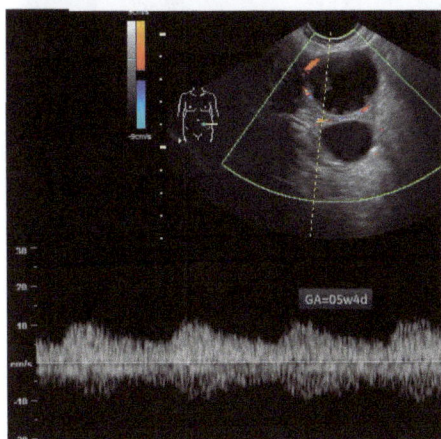

3.42h

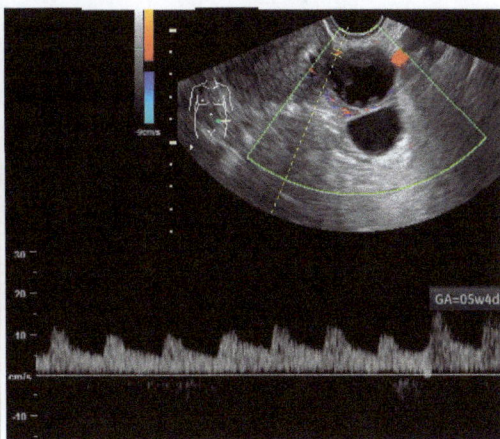

3.42i

Ultrasound report: An IUGS measuring 13 x 13 x 13mm with a YS measuring 3 x 3 x 3mm. No EP is demonstrated. No obvious ultrasound evidence or cause for pvb is demonstrated. The right ovary is measuring 32 x 23 x 25mm (9.6mls) and in it is a 15 x 14 x 15mm corpus luteum. The left ovary is measuring 56 x 56 x 34mm

(55.8mls) and in it are two septated cystic areas measuring 32 x 28 x 33mm and 26 x 21 x 25mm. The larger one of the cysts is vascular on Colour flow Dopplers and has tiny scattered echogenic areas.

Impression: An early pregnancy. Normal right ovary. Left ovarian pathology cannot be excluded and this will require appropriate follow up

3.5

This patient was referred with a history of vaginal bleeding for 3/7 and hyperemesis. GA by LMP = 15+4 at the time of the scan. The right ovary was not visualised.

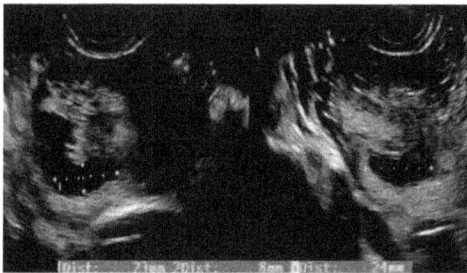
3.5a

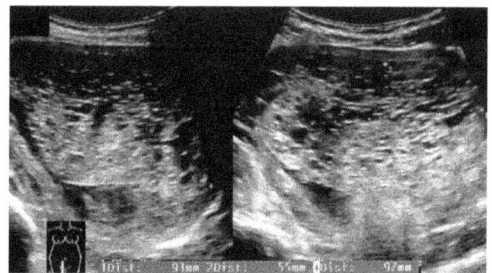
3.5b

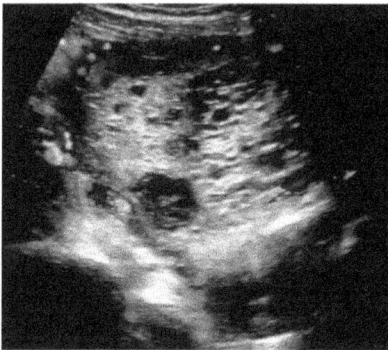
3.5c

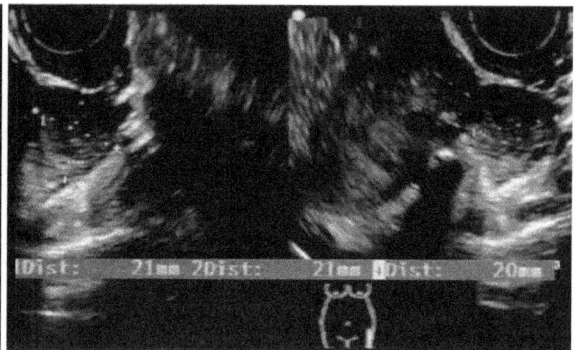
3.5d

Ultrasound findings: The uterus is filled with multicystic changes, ?grape-like appearances (3.5a–c). The largest cystic space is 23 × 24mm. No obvious yolk sac or fetal pole demonstrated. The left ovary appears normal measuring 21 × 21 × 20mm (4.6ml) 3.5d. No free fluid is seen in the POD.

Impression: Hydatidiform mole.

*Histology report confirmed a complete hydatidiform mole.

Previous bad or poor obstetric history

This group includes patients who have had a poor obstetric history or experienced conditions, such as previous ectopic pregnancy, molar pregnancy, missed abortion or miscarriage, or fetal abnormality. It is important that the sonographer finds out the nature of the bad history before commencing the scan either by liaising with the referring clinician or midwife if that information has not been supplied on the request form or by asking the patient. Details of a bad history can help to focus more on the reason for certain ultrasound findings. The sonographer should naturally expect that such a patient may attend with much anxiety and awareness of the previous obstetric ultrasound experience. As soon as the pregnancy location and fetal heartbeats are confirmed and there are no obvious abnormalities peculiar to that GA are found, the patient should be told the findings. Then the sonographer can continue the scan and complete it in line with the departmental protocol.

3.6

This patient was referred with a history of previous bad obstetric history. The findings are shown below. Both ovaries (not shown) appeared sonographically normal.

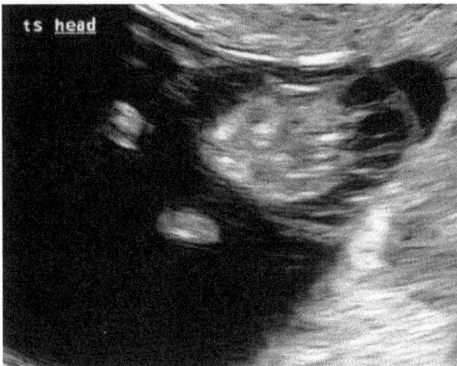 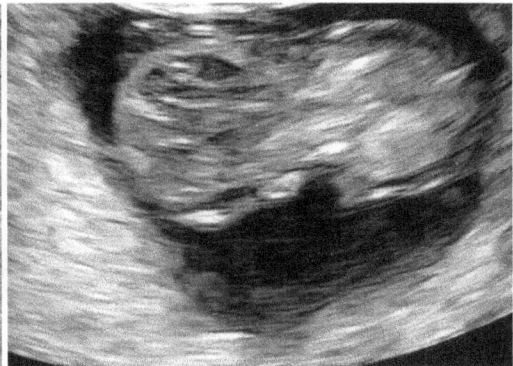

3.6a   **3.6b**

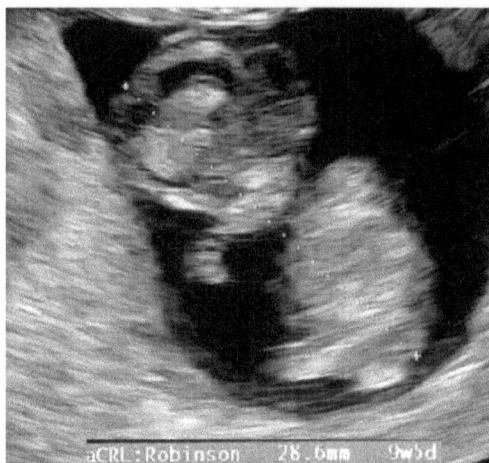

3.6c

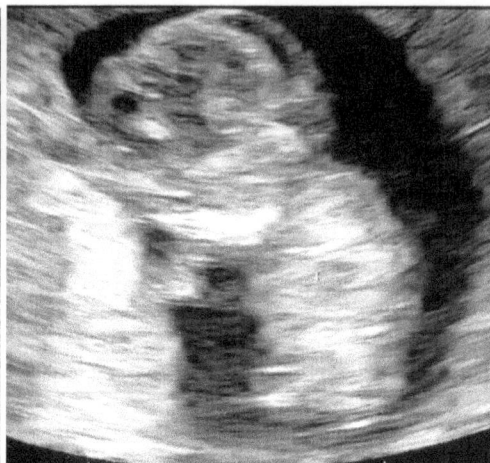

3.6d

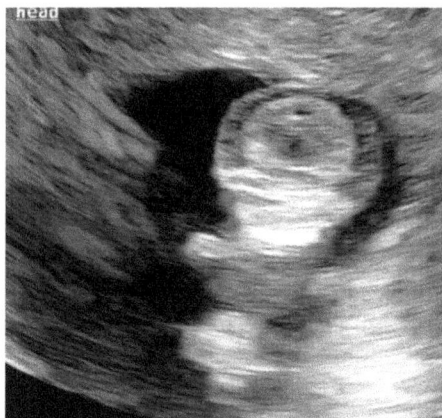

3.6e

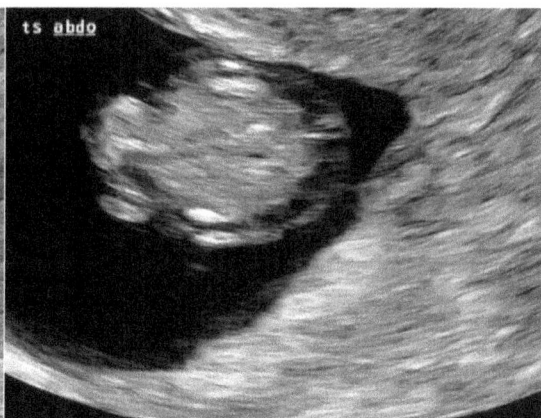

3.6f

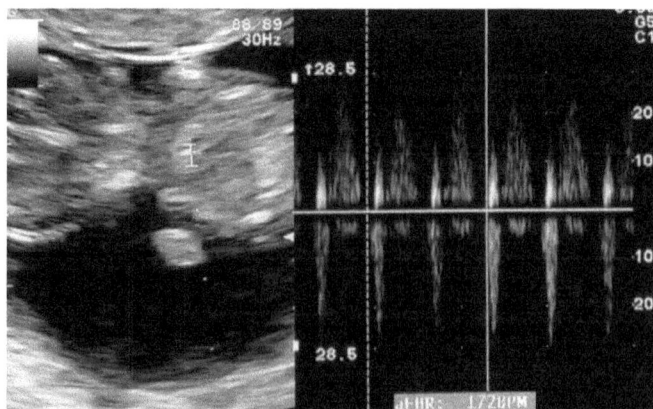

3.6g

Ultrasound findings: Single intrauterine pregnancy.

CRL = 28.6mm = 9+5/40 (3.6c). EHR = 172bpm (3.6g). There is oedema around the fetus and a septated cystic entity around the fetal head (3.6a–f).

Impression: Cystic hygroma

- Follow-up scan a few days later confirmed the diagnosis
- EHR at 13+6 /40 scan = 90bpm = severe brachycardia
- Patient is married to her first cousin.
  - There are claims that there is an increased risk of death – throughout the world – of 1.2% in children born within first-cousin marriages
  - In terms of birth defects, the risks rise from about 2% in the general population to 4% when the parents are closely related
  - Genetic conditions that are more common in populations with high rates of consanguineous marriage include rare recessive disorders, which causea wide range of problems, such as blindness, deafness, skin diseases, and neurodegenerative conditions
  - Cousin marriage is a preferred and sustained practice in many parts of the world and there are members of some communities who believe that it has significant social, economic and community benefits. However, there is a potential health risk arising from recessive genetic disorders
  - The absolute risk to first cousins having a child with a recessive genetic condition is about three in every 100 births, unless they have a family history of an autosomal recessive disorder, in which case the risk may be higher. When there is the background risk of having a child with any type of congenital or genetic disorder, which applies in every pregnancy, the overall risk for first cousins rises to about six in every 100 births, i.e. double the risk in the general population. However, most pregnancies do not result in abnormalities.

    This pregnancy ended as a second-trimester IUD. Subsequent pregnancy ended well.

Unknown or unsure LMP – dating scan

It is not uncommon for patients not to remember their LMP or to be unsure of it. For others the monthly menstrual period is irregular or shorter or longer than 28 days. Some conceive whilst taking the contraceptive pill, and this can happen if they do not take it every day or if they had to take antibiotics. Some patients bleed or have spotting at the expected time of the normal monthly period. Some patients conceive immediately following a recent miscarriage so there is no LMP, and some conceive whilst breastfeeding. Therefore, these patients may be sent for a dating scan.

3.8

This patient was referred with a clinical history of conceiving whilst breastfeeding.
LMP – Unsure

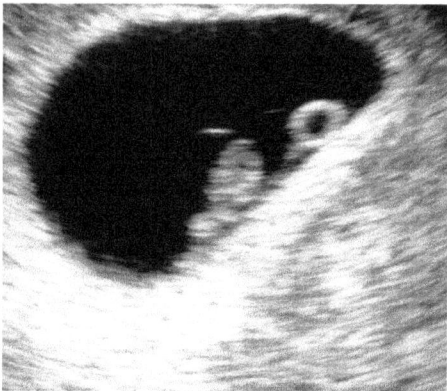

3.8a

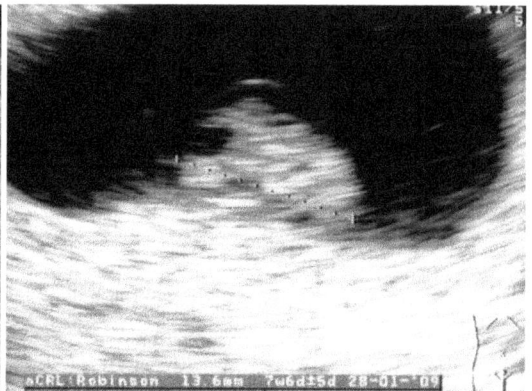

3.8b

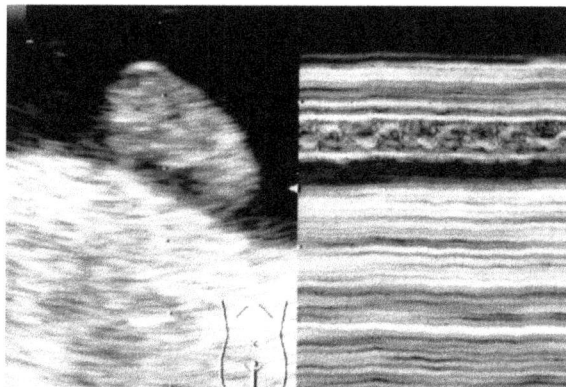

3.8c

Ultrasound findings: An IUGS, YS, FP and EHB (3.8a–c). CRL – 14mm = 7+6/40 (3.b). Pregnancy was now dated by CRL and the appropriate EDD was assigned.
Impression: Single intrauterine pregnancy.
* Breastfeeding only makes a patient less fertile but not infertile.
It is not unusual for a patient not to have a period for months after having a baby.

Her ovaries, however, may release her first post-partum egg 2 weeks before her period, making it possible for her to conceive before her first post-partum monthly period.

3.9

This patient stopped the contraceptive pill 2 months before this scan. By her LMP, GA = 10+6. She was referred for a dating scan. Both ovaries (not shown here) appeared sonographically normal.

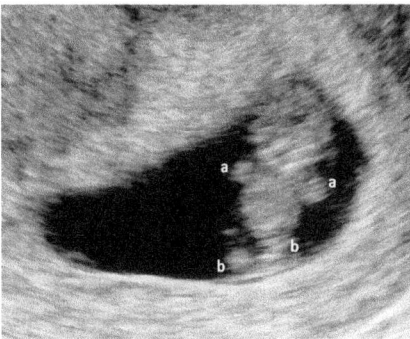 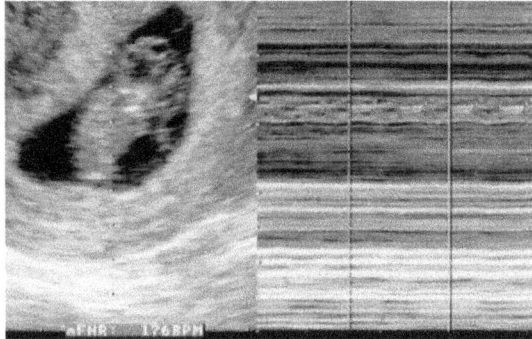

| 3.9a | 3.9b |

a- upper limb bud, b- lower limb bud

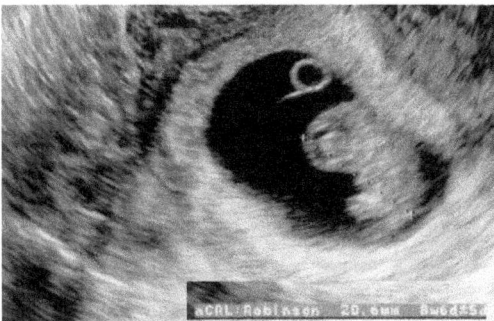 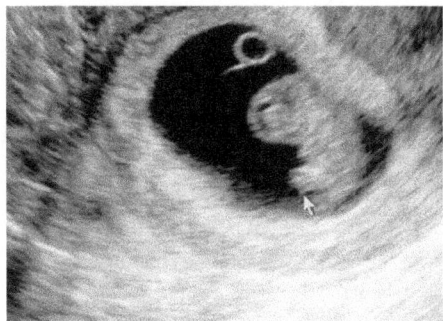

| 3.9c | 3.9d |

Ultrasound findings: Single IUP with an embryo and yolk sac (3.9a, c–d). EHB is demonstrated in 3.9b, CRL = 20.6mm = 8+6/40 (3.9c). Pregnancy has to be redated by the CRL; this will mean a new EDD has to be assigned.
Impression: Single ongoing IUP.
Note the gut herniation at the cord insertion. Arrow head. This is normal at this GA. Note the primitive limb buds just coming out in 3.9a.

3.10

This patient was referred for a scan, GA by LMP = 6+5/40. LMP - Unsure.

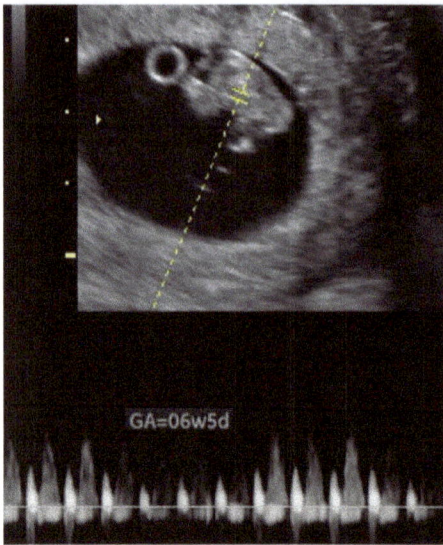

3.10a

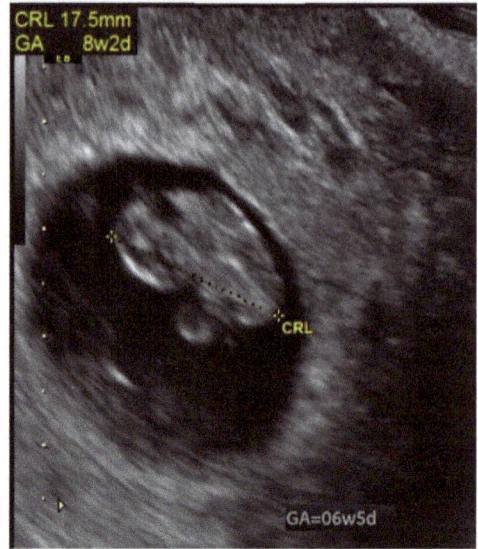

3.10b

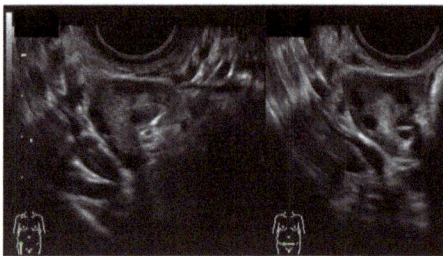

3.10c

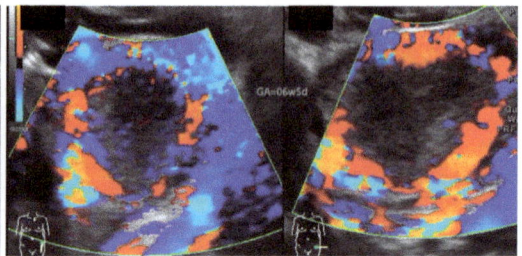

3.10d

3.10c Normal ultrasound appearances of the right ovary.

3.10d. 'Ring of fire' around the corpus luteum in the left ovary (arrow in 3.10d).

Note the 'ring of fire' around the corpus luteum in the left ovary (3.10d). It is a normal finding.

Ultrasound findings: There is an IUGS, YS, FP and EHB (3.10a–b). GA by LMP = 6+5/40, but GA by CRL is 8+2/40 (3.10b). The right ovary appears sonographically normal (3.10c) There is a corpus luteum in the left ovary (3.10d).

Impression: An ongoing pregnancy. As the pregnancy is much bigger than expected, a new EDD was assigned using the CRL.

CRL will be wrong where and when:
- The calipers are faulty
- The CRL is done after 14 weeks' GA
- The yolk sac is included in the measurement as (see image below)
- The longest length of the embryo or fetus is not measured
- The measurement is taken when the embryo or fetus is curled or

hyperextended as in the stretching out position

Below are images of the same embryo

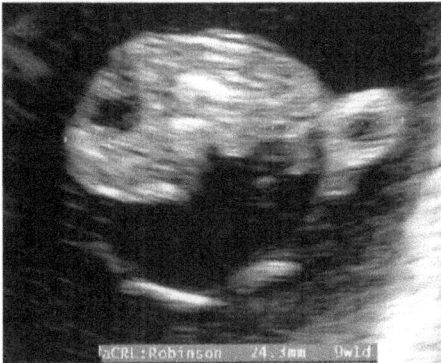

3.11a CRL = 24.3mm = 9+1/40   **3.11b** CRL = 18.5mm = 8+4/40.

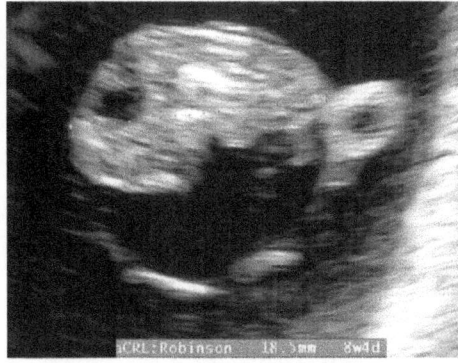

Wrong measurement in 3.11a as the yolk right is included in the CRL.
To overcome the above reasons for incorrect CRL:
- The ultrasound equipment QA tests should be performed regularly to ensure that the calipers are working accurately
- CRL is not done after 14 weeks' GA rather the HC/BPD/FL should be done and used instead for dating the pregnancy
- The yolk sac is not included in the CRL measurement
- It is not unusual not to be able to get the longest CRL measurement of the embryo or fetus at the first time. It is important that the embryo or fetus be allowed to move of his or her own accord and the sonographer record and measure the fetus in the longest natural length, i.e. without any neck extension
- Ensure that the image for the CRL is enlarged on the screen so it becomes easier to place the calipers more accurately
- In multiple pregnancies where the pregnancy is to be dated by CRL, the bigger or longer CRL should be used to date the pregnancy

Once the GA and EDD have been ascertained by ultrasound CRL, please do not change the EDD. Not changing the EDD assigned by ultrasound will:

- Ensure that tests such as the combined test and any other blood tests are carried out at the appropriate times
- Ensure the patient is booked for her other ultrasound examinations at the appropriate times
- Check that IUGR is not missed later in the pregnancy
- Ensure big babies are not missed
- Ensure obstetric deliveries are carried out at the appropriate time

3.12

This patient was referred for a dating scan. The right ovary (not shown here) appeared sonographically normal .

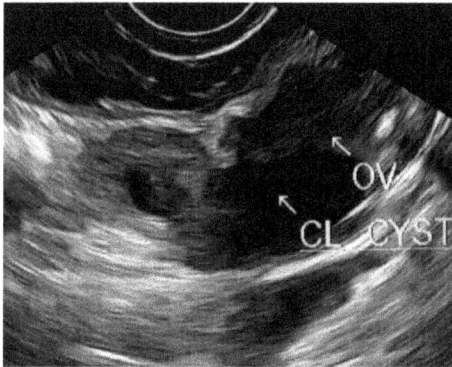

3.12a

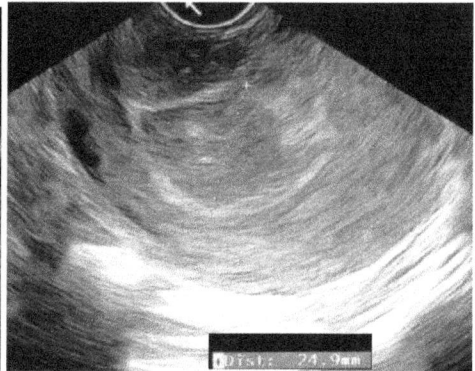

3.12b

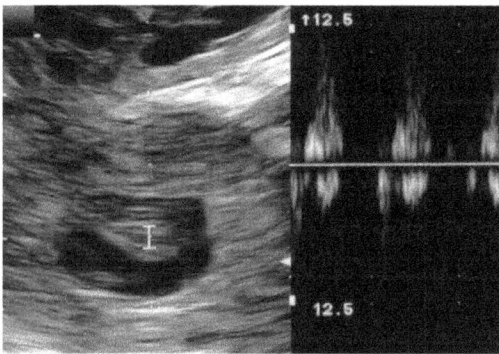

3.12c

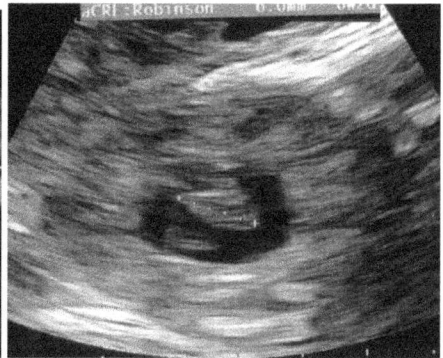

3.12d

Ultrasound findings: A retroverted uterus with a 25mm endometrium containing some low-level echoed material. No obvious IUGS is demonstrated (3.12a). There is a corpus luteum in the left ovary (3.12b). Adjacent to the left ovary is a doughnut sign or adnexal ring: GS, FP and EHB, CRL = 6mm = 6+2/40 (3.12c–d).

Impression: Unruptured live ectopic pregnancy in the left adnexa. Decidual reaction in the endometrium and a corpus luteal cyst in the left ovary.

* Diagnosis of unruptured ectopic pregnancy was confirmed at surgery.

3.13
This patient was sent for a dating scan. FHB was seen but is not shown here.

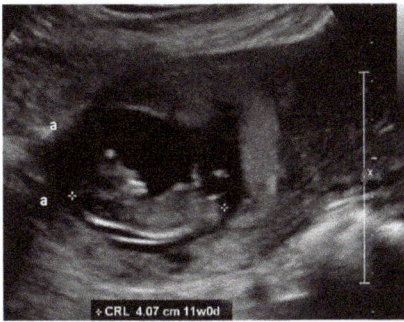 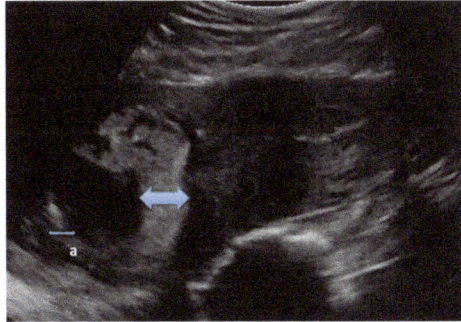

3.13a **3.13b**

TAS Views

a-shows some part of the gestational sac not completely surrounded by the myometrium

Thin arrow shows some part of the gestational sac that is not completely surrounded by the myometrium. Block arrow shows placenta and area surrounded by the myometrium

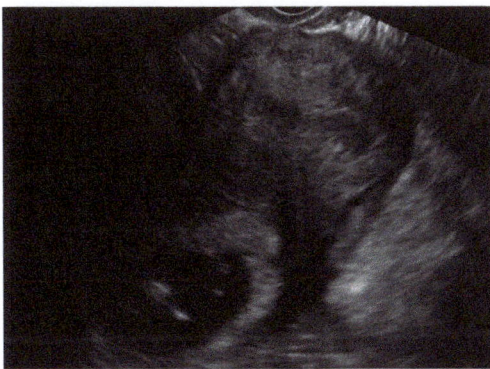 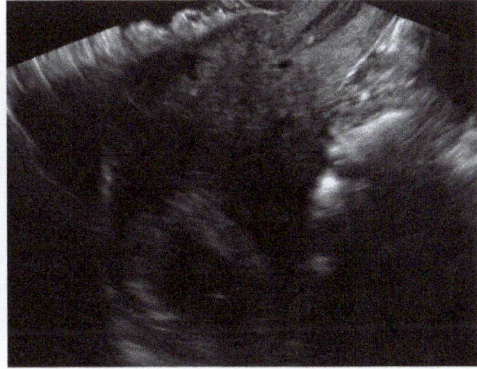

3.13d **3.13d.**

TVS Views

Ultrasound findings: Eccentrically located intrauterine pregnancy with a single fetus (3.13a–b). The myometrium does not completely surround the gestational sac (3.13a–c) see the arrows. CRL = 40.7mm = 11+0/40 (3.13a). FHB was reported as seen but not shown here.

Impression: Right cornual or interstitial pregnancy.

* Right cornual pregnancy was confirmed at surgery.

A cornual or interstitial pregnancy
- Is an ectopic pregnancy
- Is usually eccentrically positioned in the uterus
- Will have some part of the gestational sac not completely surrounded by the myometrium
- May rupture later than other tubal pregnancies – often with massive intraperitoneal hemorrhage because of the dilated arcuate artery and veins
- Represents only 2–4.7% of all ectopic pregnancies
- Risk factors include previous salpingectomy and assisted reproduction
- Cases that advance beyond 12 weeks' gestation (20%) end in rupture
- In contrast to a tubal ectopic pregnancy, which may rupture at 6–8 weeks' gestation, an interstitial ectopic pregnancy may progress without symptoms until rupture occurs at 12–16 weeks
- Maternal mortality from cornual pregnancy is quoted as twice that of other tubal pregnancies

*In the above case the patient was asymptomatic.

Previous molar pregnancy

In view of the possibility of developing another molar pregnancy an early scan is mandatory for a patient who has had a previous molar pregnancy. Such an ultrasound will help to confirm or exclude an IUP as the cause for raised levels of β-hCG, i. e. not a recurrence of a molar pregnancy.

3.14

This patient was referred for a scan at 8+3/40 with a history of previous molar pregnancy. Both ovaries (not shown) appeared sonographically normal.

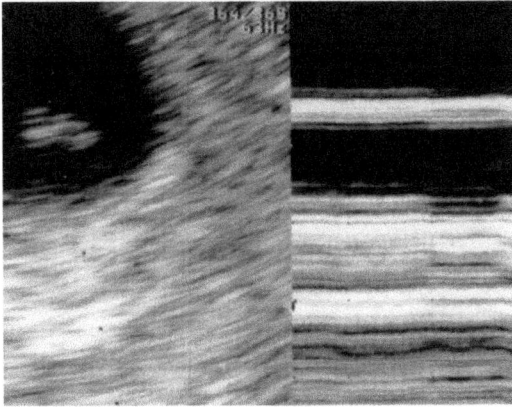 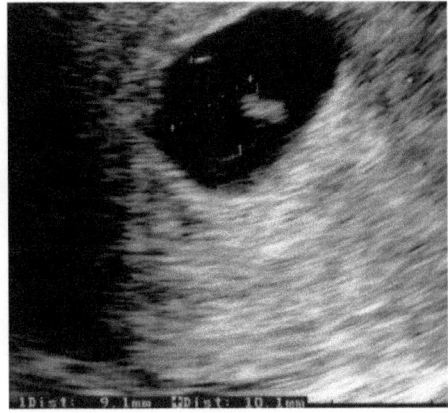

| 3.14a | 3.14b |

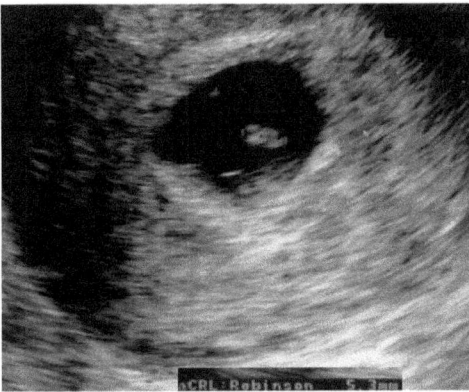 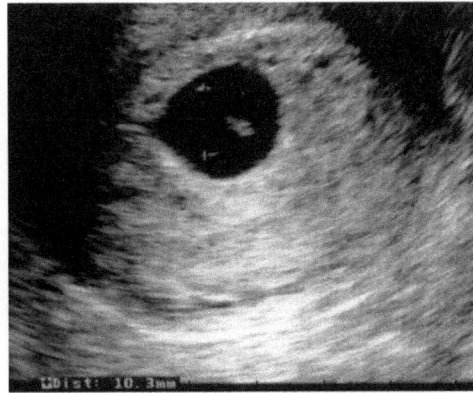

| 3.14c | 3.14d |

Ultrasound findings: A slightly irregular in outline IUGS, YS and EP (3.14b–d) but with no EHB. (3.14a). YS measurement is 10 × 9 × 10mm (3.14c–d).

Impression: The YS measurement is too large for GA. The fetal pole size does not correspond to the YS or GS size and there is no EHB (3.14a). CRL = 5.3mm = ?6+2/40 < than dates. Ultrasound appearances are that of a missed abortion or miscarriage (MA).

In line with the RCOG guideline, findings will have to be confirmed with another Sonographer or Obstetrician. A follow up scan 7-10days later may be arranged depending on the departmental protocol.

3.15

This patient was referred for a scan at 8+/40 with a history of maternal anxiety and previous molar pregnancy. The right ovary was not identified.

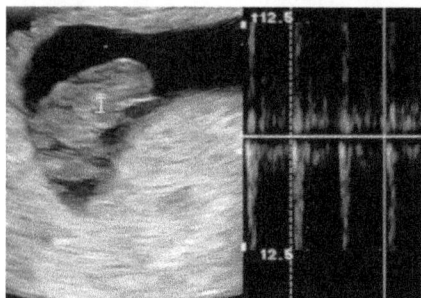 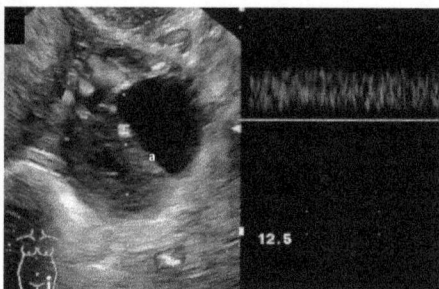

3.15a	**3.15b**

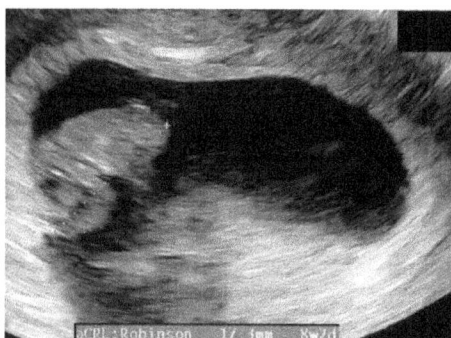 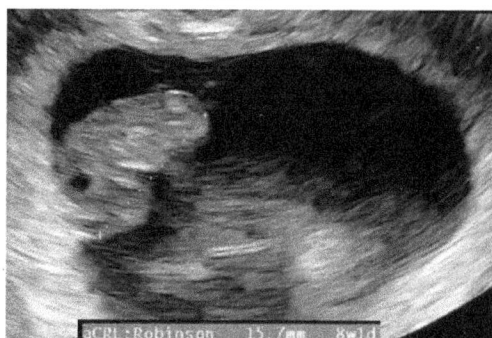

3.15c	**3.15d**

Ultrasound findings: Single IUP and EHB demonstrated (3.15a, c–d). CRL = 17.3mm = 8+2/40. (3.15c). There is a cyst with a vascular component on the left – ? retracting clot with a horizontal level and clear serum compone nt, ? cyst with fluid-debris level (3.15b).

Impression: Ongoing pregnancy. Cyst in the left maternal adnexa.

The left ovary should be assessed at a subsequent ultrasound examination.

Previous ectopic pregnancy

Patients who have had an ectopic pregnancy are prone to a recurrence in another pregnancy. It is good practice to scan these patients early in the subsequent pregnancy to confirm or otherwise the location of the pregnancy and date it.

3.16

This patient was referred at 7+3/40 with a history of previous ectopic pregnancy.

Right ovary (not shown here) appeared sonographically normal.

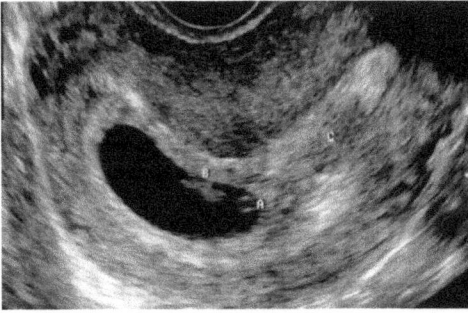

3.16a

3.16a - a – YS, b – EP.

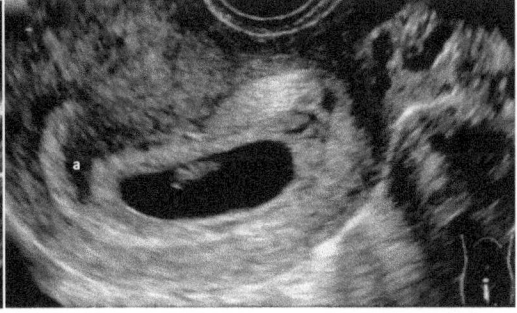

3.16b

3.16b- a-?implantational bleed

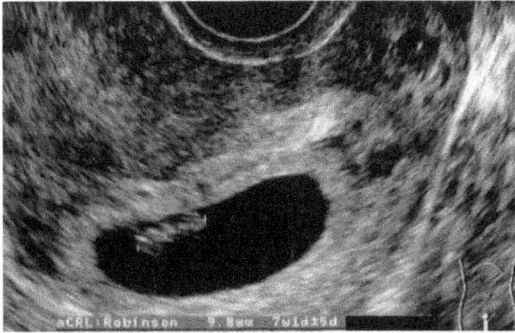

3.16c

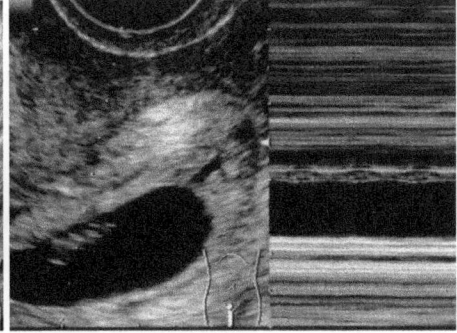

3.16d

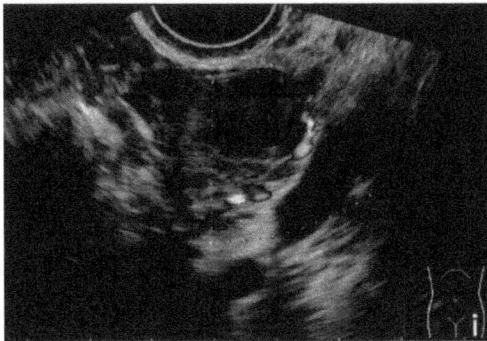

3.16e

Ultrasound findings: An IUGS with a YS, EP (3.16a–c) and EHB (3.16d). CRL = 9.8mm = 7+1/40 (3.16c). There is a corpus luteum in the left ovary (3.16e). There is a small hypoechoic area superior to the GS. ? implantational bleed (3.16b).

Impression: Ongoing IUP.

* These findings are very reassuring for the patient and her pregnancy can be monitored according to the hospital policy or protocol.

3.17

This patient was referred with a history of previous ectopic pregnancy and maternal anxiety. This was a natural conception. EHB (not shown here) was present

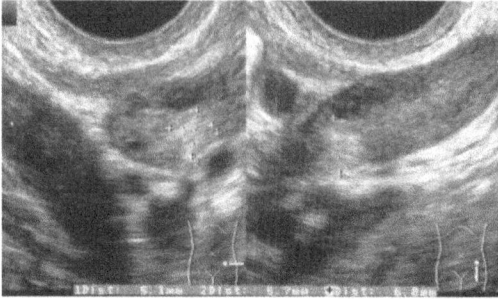
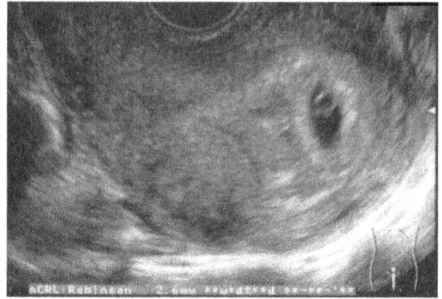

3.17a   **3.17b**

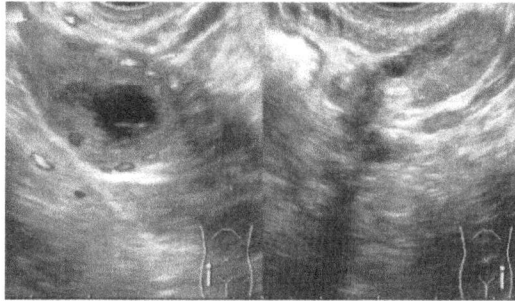

3.17c

Ultrasound findings: Retroverted uterus with an intrauterine gestational sac, yolk sac, embryonic pole. CRL = 2.6mm. (3.17b) In the right ovary is a corpus luteum (3.17c – first half of the image). This is a normal finding. There is an approx. 5 × 6 × 7mm echogenic area in the left ovary (3.17a and second half of 3.17c arrow). This is probably a dermoid cyst. The right ovary appears sonographically normal and in it is a corpus luteum (3.17c first °°half of the image).

Impression: Single intrauterine gestational pregnancy. Normal ultrasound appearances of the right ovary. There is probably a dermoid cyst in the left ovary.

Fertility treatments and ultrasound scanning

Patients who conceive by fertility treatment may need to be scanned to confirm the location of the pregnancy, the number of embryos or fetuses. The scan is also to confirm or refute any pregnancy-related complications as in any other normally conceived pregnancy, and fertility treatment-related complications including ovarian hyperstimulation syndrome (OHSS). These patients are generally more prone to ectopic pregnancy. Finding an intrauterine pregnancy cannot exclude a co-existing heterotopic pregnancy, especially in patients who conceive with fertility treatment and who had more than one embryo transfer in the particular treatment cycle.

Seeing multiple corpus luteal cysts and enlarged ovary or ovaries is often the clue that prompt the sonographer to ask if a pregnancy was achieved by fertility treatment as often patients may not easily provide this information. The condition OHSS may be seen in association with drug therapy used for fertility treatment. The sonographer should scan the abdomen to exclude the presence of ascites and pleural effusion when there is free fluid in the pelvis.

3.18

This patient was referred because of pain and nausea.

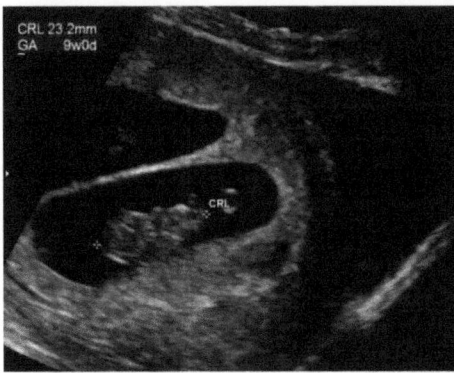

3.18a   **3.18b**

Note the lambda sign

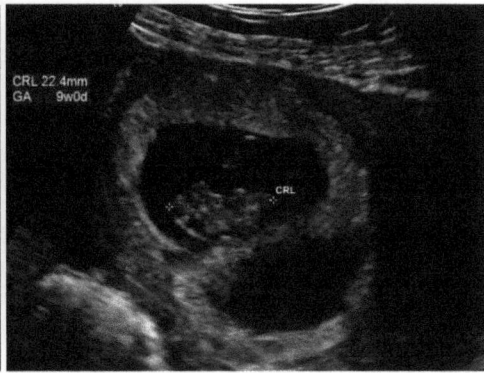

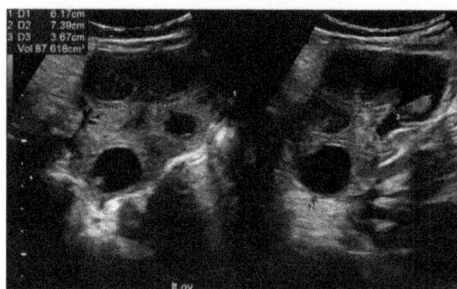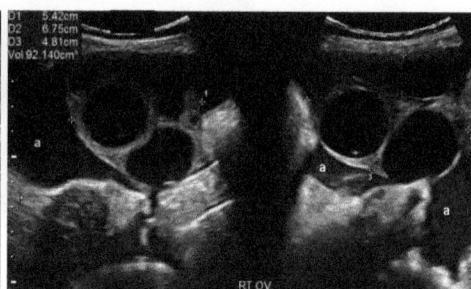

3.18c   **3.18d**

c. Note the enlarged ovaries, multiple corpus luteal cysts (3.18c–d) and a-pockets of low level echoed fluid around the right ovary

Ultrasound findings: DA/DC twins (3.18a–b). Enlarged ovaries, multiple corpus luteal cysts (3.18c–d) and low-level echoed fluid adjacent and inferior to the right ovary (3.18d).

Impression: Moderate ovarian OHSS. This was an IVF pregnancy.

Ovarian hyperstimulation syndrome (OHSS)

OHSS usually presents after egg collection and embryo transfer have taken place In fact, 75% of patients who develop OHSS are pregnant

There are three grades of OHSS

- Mild OHSS (the incidence is thought to be 8–23%); presents as elevated hormone levels and enlarged ovaries on ultrasound.
- Moderate OHSS (the incidence is 3 -6%); presentation is as in mild OHSS plus abdominal distension, nausea, vomiting and diarrhoea.
- Severe OHSS (incidence is 0.2 - 1%); presentation is as in mild OHSS plus ascites, which causes abdominal pain and distension. There is pleural effusion which causes shortness of breath, alteration in blood clotting with eventual problems with clot formation and, if untreated, reduced blood flow to the kidneys leading to reduced urine output and renal failure.
- OHSS can be life-threatening.

3.19
This patient was referred for a scan post-IVF treatment.

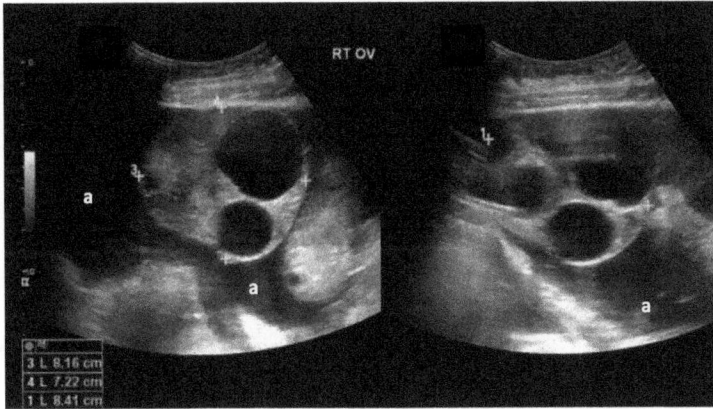

3.19a
a-pockets of low level echoed fluid around the right ovary

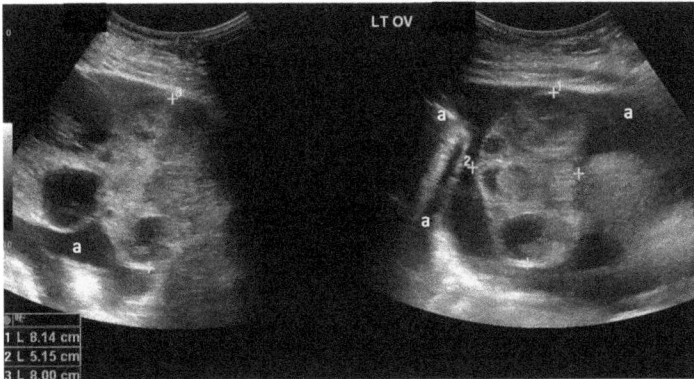

3.19b
a-pockets of low level echoed fluid around the left ovary

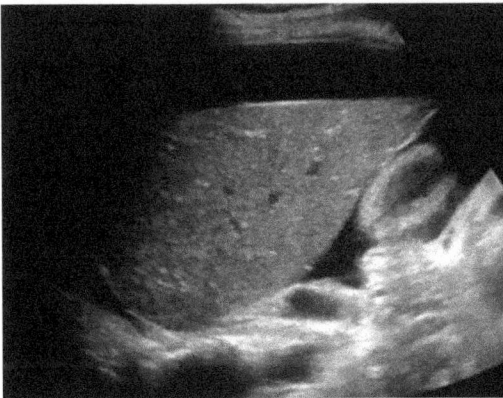

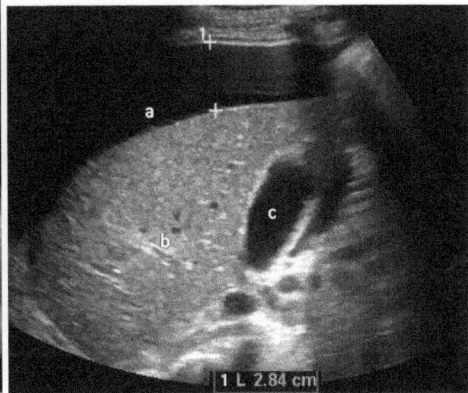

3.19c   **3.19d** *a-ascites, b-liver, c- gall bladder*

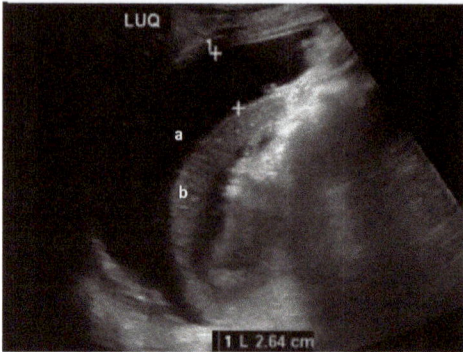

3.19e

a-ascites, b-spleen

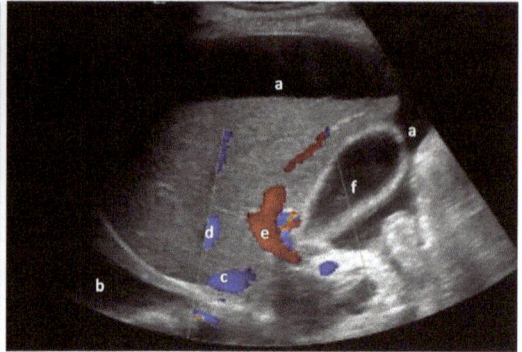

3.19f

a-ascites, b-right pleural effusion, c- IVC, d-hepatic vein, e-portal vein, f-distended gall bladder

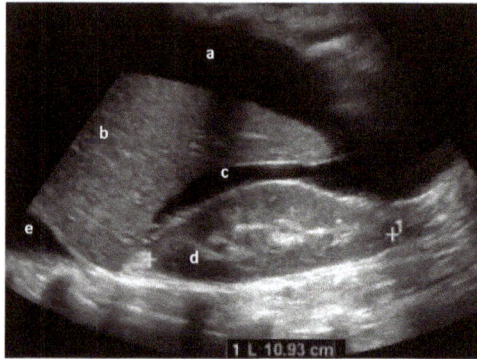

3.19g

a-ascites, b-liver, c- fluid in Morrison's pouch, d-right kidney, e – right pleural effusion

Ultrasound findings: There is gross ascites in the abdomen and pelvis. Both ovaries are enlarged with multiple corpus luteal cysts (3.19a–b). Patent hepatic and portal veins (3.19f). Bilateral pleural effusions are demonstrated (3.19c–g).

* The most likely reason for checking the portal and hepatic veins is – the hallmark of OHSS is the increased vascular permeability with haemo concentration. As a result the patient is in a hypercoagulable state and is likely to develop venous thrombosis.

2 days later

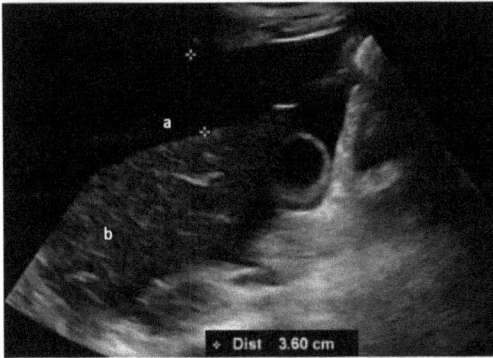

3.20a

a-ascites, b - liver

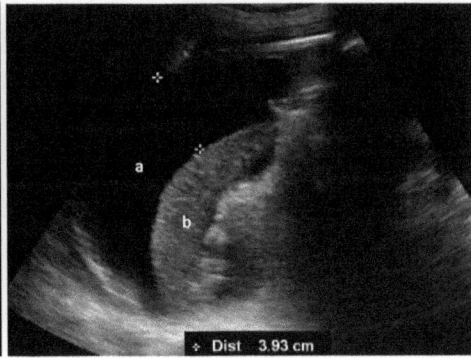

3.20b

a-ascites, b-spleen

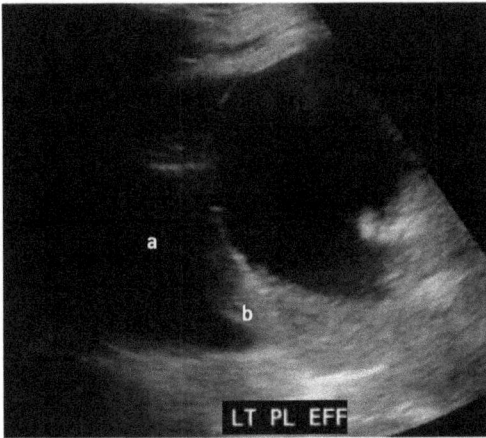

3.20c
a-left pleural effusion, b-spleen

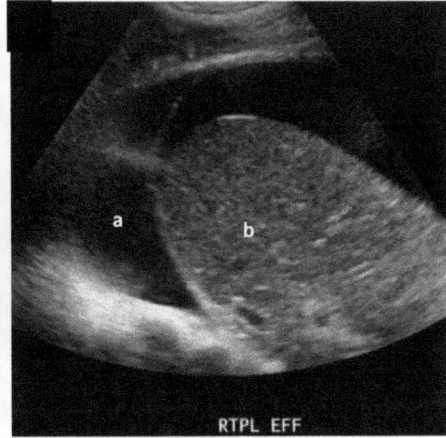

3.20d
a- right plueral effusion. c-liver

Compared with the initial scan there is an increase in the ascites and pleural effusions (compare 3.19e with 3.20b).

The patient had an ultrasound-guided drain inserted.

3.21

20 days after the initial scan

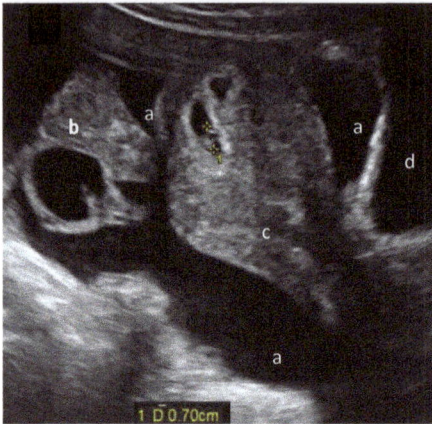
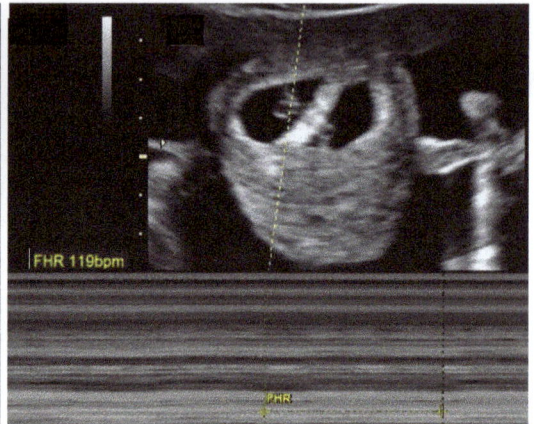

3.21a   **3.21b**

a-ascites, b-right ovary, c-gravid uterus, d-maternal urinary bladder

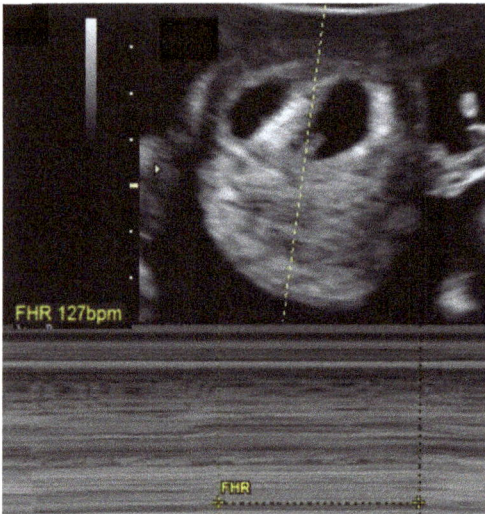
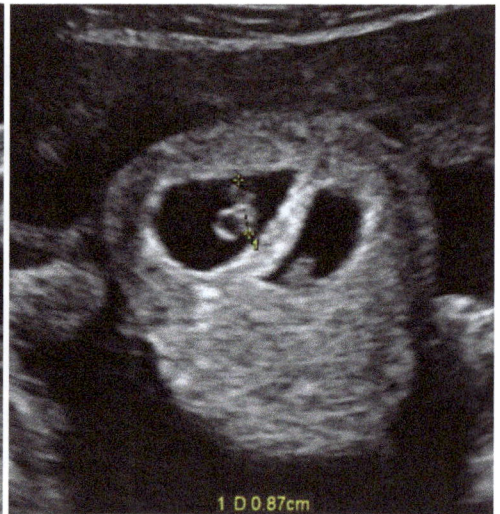

3.21c   **3.21d**

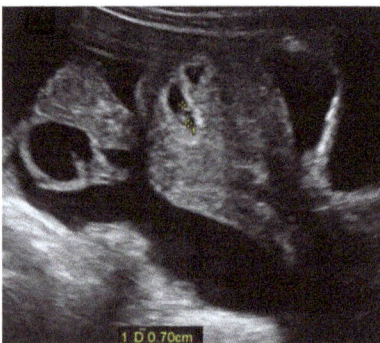
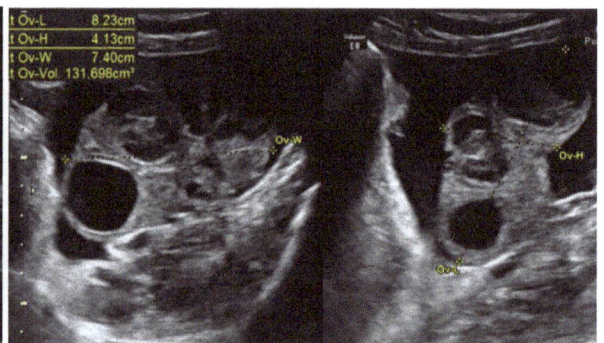

3.21e   **3.21f**

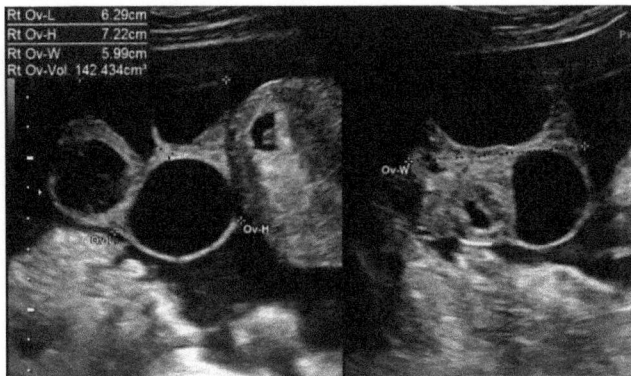

3.21g

Ultrasound findings; There is a DC/DA twin pregnancy with yolk sacs, embryos poles and EHBs. CRLs – 7mm and 8.7mm (3.21a–e). Both ovaries are still enlarged, left ovarian volume = 132ml and the right ovarian volume = 142ml. (3.21f–g). There is ascites in the pelvis (3.21a–g).

Impression: Twin pregnancy and severe OHSS.

The patient will need continuous ultrasound monitoring of the ascites and pregnancy according to departmental protocols

The above is an example of severe OHSS.

Diagnosed multiple pregnancies should be noted on further scan requests so that double scheduled appointment time-slots can be assigned to the patient.

3.22

This patient was referred because of vaginal bleeding and maternal anxiety 18 days post-one embryo transfer. Pregnancy was achieved by ovum donation.

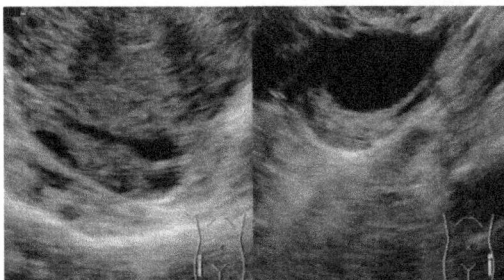
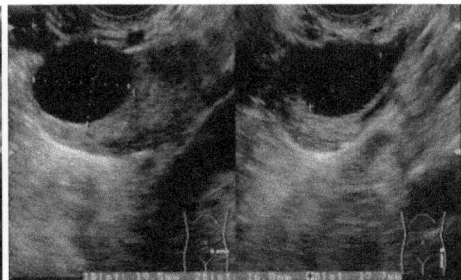

3.22a   3.22b

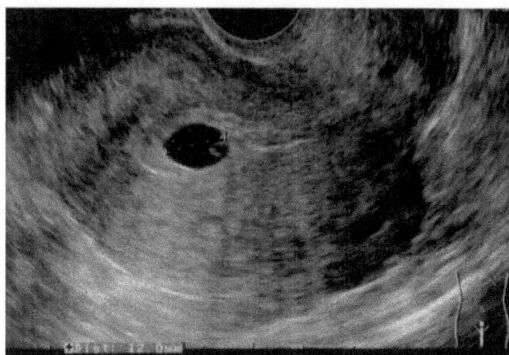 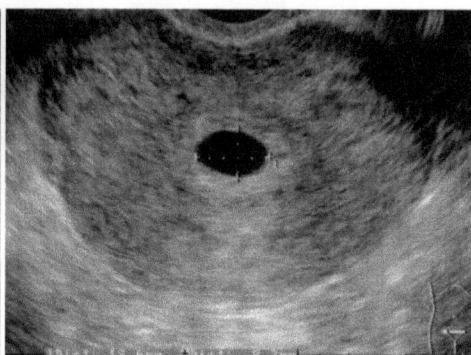

3.22c   **3.22d**

Ultrasound findings: There is an intrauterine gestational sac measuring 12 × 13 × 8mm (3.22c–d). There is a yolk sac (3.22c). There is a 18 × 16 × 20mm cyst in the left ovary (3.22b and 3.22a second part) and the right ovary appears normal (3.22a the first half of the image).

Impression: An intrauterine pregnancy.
- A follow-up scan was suggested for 7–10 days later
- OHSS is not associated with the ovum donation recipient as a patient's (receiving the embryos) ovaries are not hyperstimulated. Only her endometrium is prepared to receive the fertilised egg
- This pregnancy should be dated using the embryo transfer date not the LMP
- Should this patient opt for the combined screening test at the NT screening test later in her pregnancy, the age of the donor will be used in calculating the risk of Down's syndrome not hers

3.23
This patient, according to her IVF treatment, should be 7/40. This was her second follow-up scan. She was referred with the history of abdominal and lower back pain, no vaginal bleed, no urinary or bowel problems. Previous scan showed an empty IUGS.

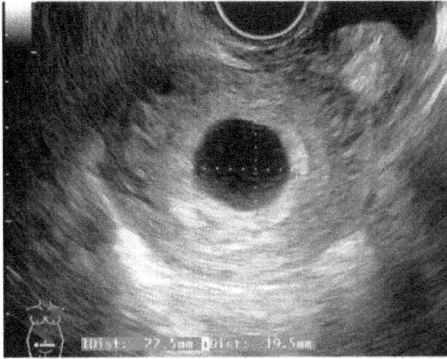

3.23a

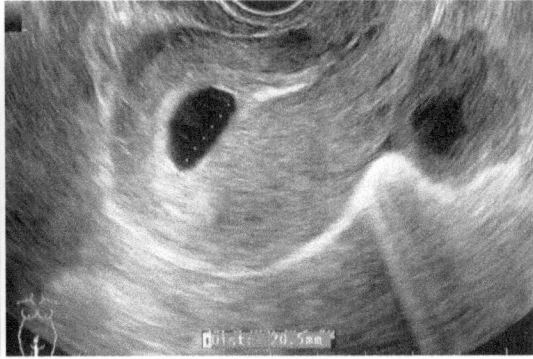

3.23b

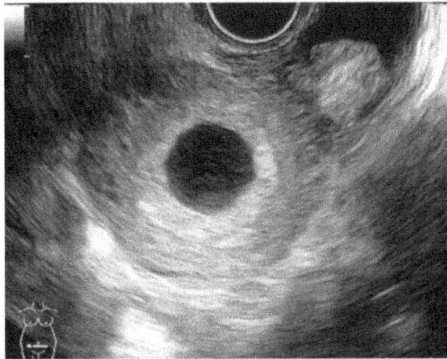

3.23c

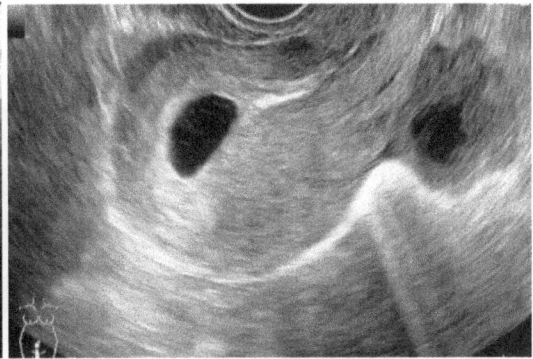

3.23d

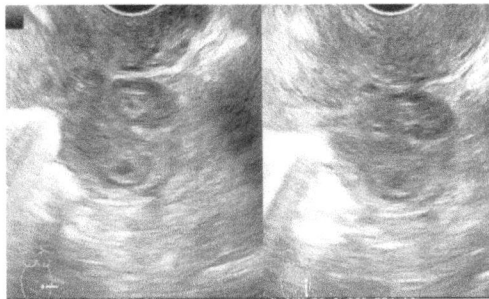

3.23e

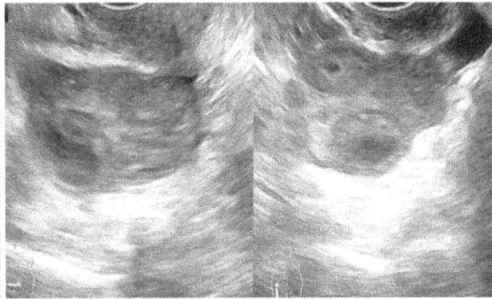

3.23f

Ultrasound findings: There is an IUGS measuring approx. 21 × 23 × 20mm (3.23a–d). No obvious YS or embryonic pole has been demonstrated. GSV = 2.1 × 2.3 × 2 cm × 0.5233 = 5.06 ml. Both ovaries are enlarged and multiple cysts are demonstrated in them (3.23e–f). There is some fluid in the POD (3.23d)

Impression: Blighted ovum or an embryonic pregnancy. Bilateral enlarged ovaries with multiple cysts.

* With IVF, the GA is certain as this is calculated from the embryo transfer date. Previous scan was reported as showing an empty IUGS.

At 7/40, normally a YS and embryonic pole should be seen in a normal ongoing pregnancy. Equally with the GSV of 5.06 ml, a YS and embryonic pole should be seen. Therefore, one can say with confidence that it is a blighted ovum or an anembryonic pregnancy.

* IVF pregnancies are also subjective to all the complications as seen in any normally conceived pregnancy.

Clomid treatment

Fertility treatment with clomifene (Clomid) is aimed at helping the patient to produce not more than three eggs in one menstrual cycle. Clomid treatment is often used as the first step in treating infertility where there are no suspicions of Fallopian tube problems. The patient is prescribed some Clomid tablets which she takes from day 2 to day 6 of her cycle or from day 1 to day 5. Clomid tablets are given in 50mg or its multiples. The starting dose is usually 50mg and if that does not work, the dose can be increased to 100mg or 150mg in the next treatment cycles. The increased dose may boost her ability to produce one but not more than three eggs. Ideally the patient is scanned at day 10 to monitor the endometrium and ovaries. Subsequent scans in the cycle will depend on the ultrasound findings on day 10. Once the dominant follicle has reached the desired size, an injection is given to trigger the egg release and the patient is advised to have sexual intercourse. Where more than three follicles are growing and are likely to become large enough to produce ova, the patient will be advised not to have intercourse in that cycle until after her next period as she is considered prone to hyperstimulation and to multiple pregnancy. Mature follicular size is between 14 and 23mm but may be up to 30mm when the ovary is stimulated.

Patients who are suitable for Clomid treatment are those who can produce their own natural follicles, have not had any tubal problems or previous tubal surgery, preferably without any history of PID or any sexually transmitted disease to prevent ectopic pregnancies. Unlike IVF treatment, with Clomid treatment, there is no need to harvest the eggs in the operating theatre, no need for injections to boast multiple follicular growth, and no need for embyo transfer. The patient is advised when it is appropriate to cohabit with her husband or partner naturally.

3.24

This patient was referred for a scan at 6+5/40 following Clomid plus tamoxifen treatment with a history of LIF pain.

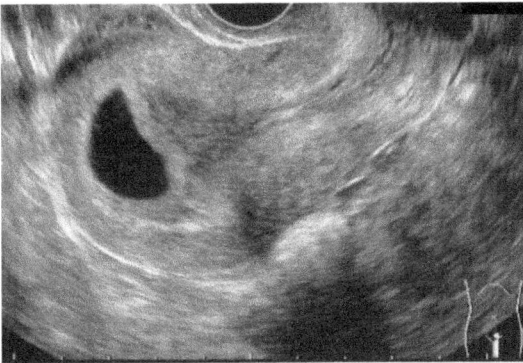

3.24a

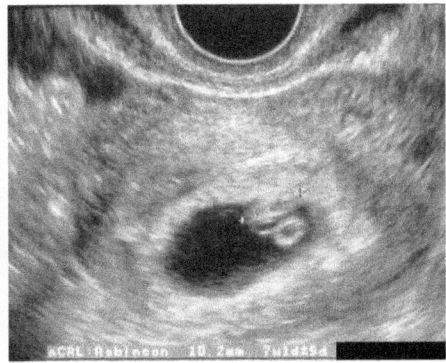

3.24b

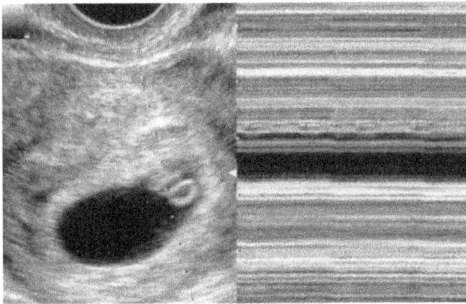

3.24c

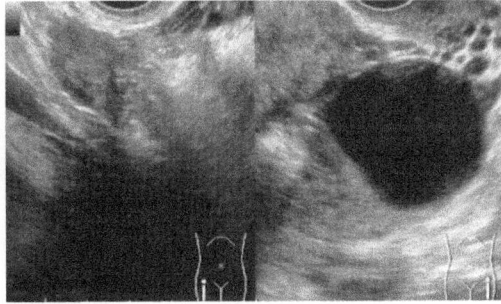

3.24d

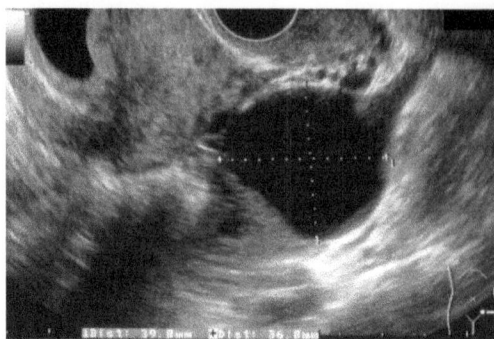 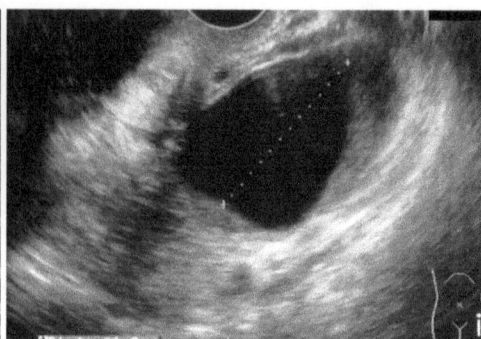

| 3.24e | 3.24f |

Ultrasound findings. An IUP, YS, embryonic pole (3.24a, b) and EHB (3.24c). CRL =10.2mm= 7+1/40 (3.24b). There is a 42 × 40 × 37mm corpus luteum in the left ovary (3.24e–f) and the second half of (3.24d). Right ovary as shown appears sonographically normal (3.24d first half of the image).

Impression: Single ongoing intrauterine pregnancy. Corpus luteum in the left ovary. Right ovary appears normal.

Tamoxifen is sometimes used in patients who experience failure to ovulate or conceive with the use of clomiphene. Some experts believe that tamoxifen is a good first-line as well as second-line ovulation-inducing agent. With tamoxifen use, all pregnancies are single with no possibility of hyperstimulation or any drug induced side-effects.

Recurrent or recent miscarriage

A spontaneous loss of a pregnancy between the time of conception and 24 weeks' gestation is termed miscarriage. These patients often attend for scanning in a state of worry, anxiety and nervous tension and sometimes they are not too hopeful of the current pregnancy. The events of the previous miscarriage(s) may still be very real and may make them tearful and very sensitive. An understanding and good tender loving care (TLC) approach by the ultrasonographer is usually appreciated and is encouraged.

Miscarriage is defined as the spontaneous loss of pregnancy before the fetus reaches viability. It should be noted that advances in neonatal care have resulted in a small number of babies surviving birth before 24 weeks' gestation. Recurrent miscarriage, defined as the loss of three or more consecutive pregnancies, affects 1% of couples trying to conceive. It has been estimated that 1–2% of second-trimester pregnancies miscarry before 24 weeks' gestation.

It is essential that a pelvic ultrasound examination with 3-D facilities, if available, be performed an all patients who experience recurrent first-trimester or second-trimester miscarriage. This is to exclude all possible ultrasound identifiable anatomic abnormalities. Such patients may also need further investigations with the use of laparoscopy or hysteroscopy to confirm or refute associated anatomical abnormalities.

3.25
This patient was referred with a history of 4 days of light bleeding and maternal anxiety. This was her fourth pregnancy but she has had three previous miscarriages under 15 weeks' gestation. GA by LMP = 7+2/40. Both ovaries (not shown here) appear sonographically normal with no obvious corpus luteum seen in them.

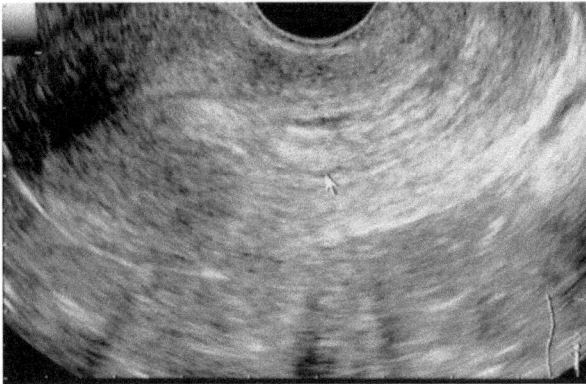

3.25a

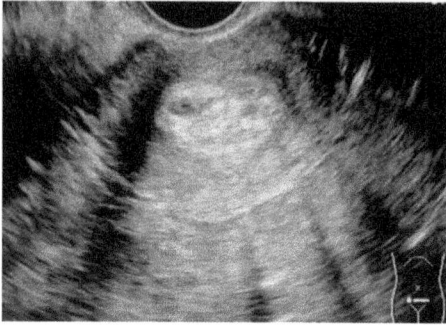 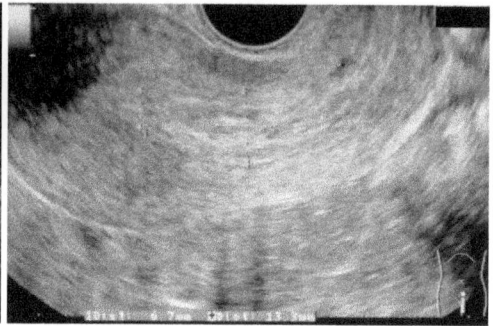

| **3.25b** | **3.25c** |

Ultrasound findings: No obvious IUGS is demonstrated. Inferior to the uterine fundus is a collection with predominantly echogenic material.

Impression: Ongoing miscarriage.
* With no obvious corpus luteum in either of the ovaries, corpus luteal defect will need to be excluded amongst other reasons or factors for miscarriage.

3.26

This patient was referred with a history of previous miscarriage and maternal anxiety. The left ovary was not visualised. FHB and movements were seen.

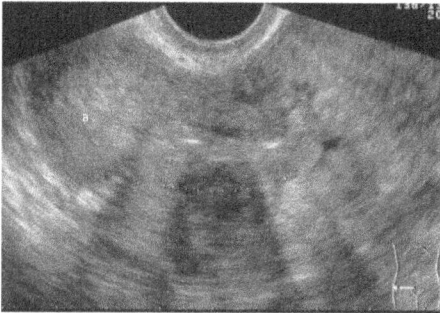 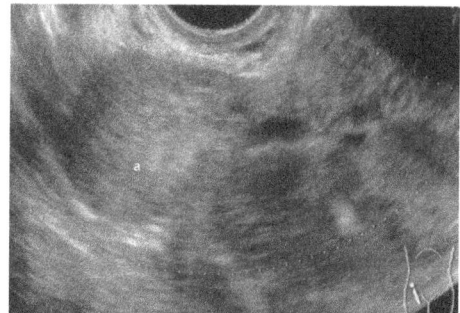

| **3.26a** | **3.26b** |

a-rudimentary horn

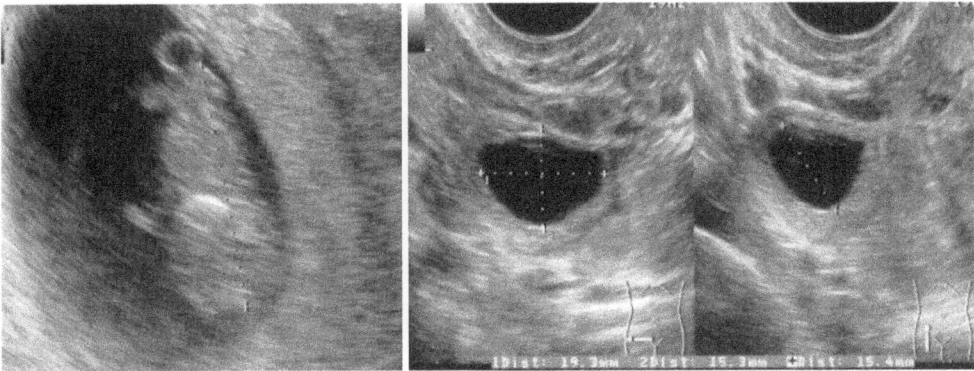

3.26c   **3.26d**

Ultrasound findings: Single intrauterine pregnancy (3.26c). CRL = 29.1mm = 9+6/40 (3.26c). Superior to the right ovary is a rudimentary horn (3.26a–b). There is a 19 × 15 × 15mm cyst in the right ovary)

Impression: Single intrauterine pregnancy in a unicornuate uterus with a rudimentary horn. There is a 19 × 15 × 15mm cyst in the right ovary.

Unicornuate uterus with a rudimentary horn is a Mullerian duct malformation
Estimated occurrence is about 1:4000
Patients with a unicornuate uterus have some of the following:
- one cervix and one vagina
- about 50% will deliver a live baby
- are prone to miscarriage, preterm delivery and IUD
- a small percentage are prone to having ectopic pregnancy
- are at higher risk of pregnancy loss and obstetrics complications

A scan of the maternal kidneys should be performed to exclude a renal abnormality as this can be an associated defect

Some causes of miscarriages

Early miscarriage	Late miscarriage	Comments
Luteal phase defect or hormonal problems	Incompetent cervix	

Up to 13/40	After 13–24/40	
Structural abnormalities of the uterus, e.g. bicornuate or unicornuate uterus	Infections, e.g. bad UTI[i], CMV[ii], HIV[iii], STDs[iv] including chlamydia, gonorrhoea and syphilis, malaria, rubella, toxoplasmosis	
Congenital fetal abnormality, e.g. trisomy 13/18 or chromosomal problems	Congenital abnormality, e.g. renal agenesis	
	Following invasive procedures such as CVS[v] or amniocentesis which both carry a 1% abortion post-either procedure	
IUCD in situ with pregnancy.	SROM or PROM[vi]	
Increased maternal age	Fibroids	Experts claim that in patients over 45 the rate of miscarriage is more than 50%. In patients 35–39, 1 in 5 (20%) will miscarry, whilst in patients under 30, 1 in 10 (10%) will miscarry
Smoking in pregnancy	PCOS[vii]	
Obesity	Hyperprolactinaemia antibodies	
Drug misuse especially cocaine	Certain medications including some drugs used for pain and arthritis, eczema and acne	

Drinking more than 2 units of alcohol per week		
Placental problems	Bacterial vaginosis	
	Long-term maternal illness/disease including hypo or hyperthyroidism, kidney problems, lupus, uncontrolled diabetes, severe high blood pressure and coeliac disease	

[i] urinary-tract infection; [ii] cytomegalovirus; [iii] human immunodeficiency virus; [iv] sexually transmitted diseases; [v] chorionic villus sampling; [vi] spontaneous rupture of membranes; [vii] polycystic ovary syndrome.

It is obvious that ultrasound cannot be used to identify many of the causes listed above

Intrauterine contraceptive devices and positive pregnancy tests

Most (if not all) patients with an IUCD in situ do not want any more pregnancies or babies. Patients who have a positive pregnancy test with a IUCD in situ may not be overly excited about the pregnancy. There is also a lurking concern of how an IUCD may affect the pregnancy should they want to proceed with the pregnancy. Apart from confirming or otherwise the location and GA of the pregnancy, the location of the IUCD if seen should be documented in relation to the pregnancy.

3.27

This patient was referred for a scan with a clinical history of positive pregnancy test result with known IUCD in situ. Both ovaries (not shown) appeared sonographically normal. FHB was seen.

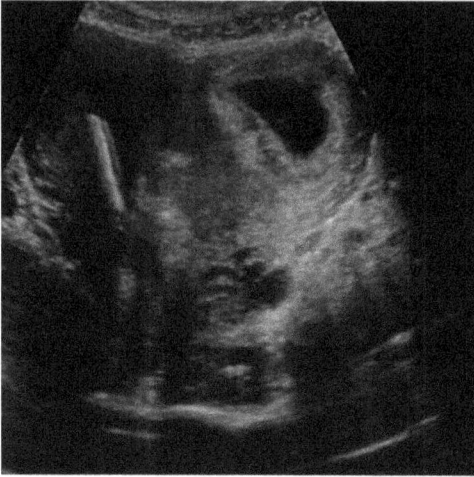 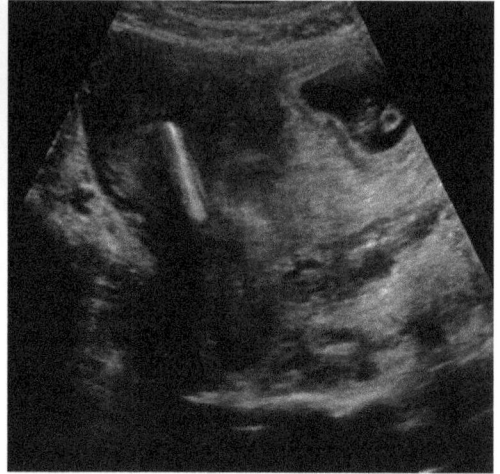

3.27a   **3.27b**

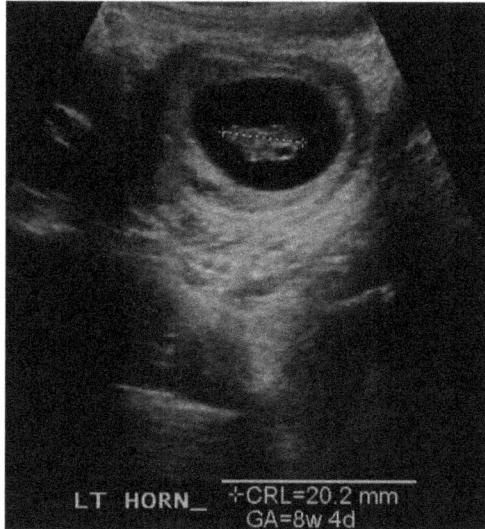

3.27c

Ultrasound findings: Bicornuate uterus with an IUGS, YS and embryonic pole seen in the left horn (3.27a–b). CRL = 20.2mm = 8+4/40 (3.27c). There is an IUCD in the right horn of the uterus (3.27a–b). This patient was not aware she had a bicornuate uterus until then.

Impression: Bicornuate uterus with the pregnancy in the left horn. IUCD is in the right horn of the uterus.

- A bicornuate uterus is an anatomical anomaly where two 'horns' are shaped at the top of the uterus forming a heart-like structure

- It occurs in about 1% of patients and often goes undiagnosed as there are often no symptoms. Spontaneous abortion is more common in patients with this condition
- This patient's kidneys should be scanned to exclude any congenital abnormality of her kidneys
- An IUCD is a small T-shaped device that is inserted into the uterus to prevent pregnancy. An IUCD is a very effective form of birth control as it can be inserted and left for 5–10 years depending on the type of IUCD. However, it is contraindicated in a patient who has a bicornuate uterus. The reason for this is because the IUCD would be inserted into only one horn of the uterus in most cases making it possible for a fertilised egg to still be able to implant in the other horn resulting in an unintended pregnancy as in this case.

3.28

This patient was referred with a positive pregnancy test result. She was known to have an IUCD in situ.

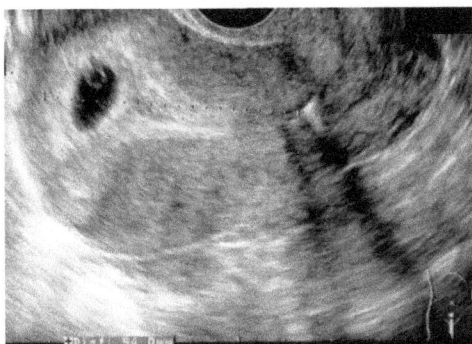
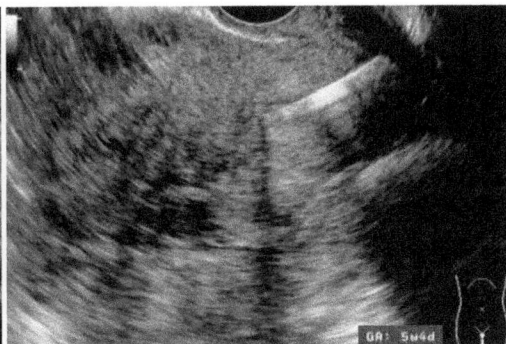

3.28a   **3.28b**

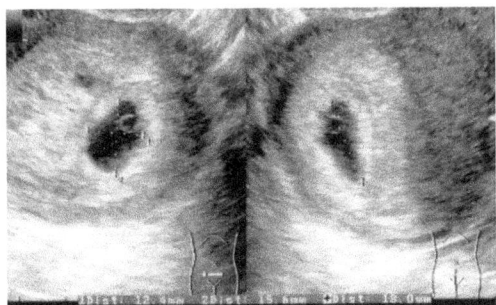
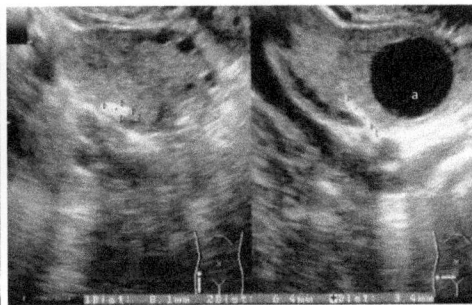

3.28c   **3.28d**

a-cyst, b -linear echogenic focus

Ultrasound findings: There is an intrauterine gestational sac measuring approx. 12 × 16 × 10mm. There is a YS but no fetal pole yet (3.28a & c). There is an IUCD in the cervical canal approx. 54mm from the uterine fundus (3.28a–b). There is an approx. 8 × 6 × 3mm linear echogenic focus as well as a cyst in the right ovary (3.28d).

Impression: There is an IUCD in the cervical canal inferior to the gestational sac. There is an echogenic focus in the right ovary

- The incidence of pregnancy with IUCDs in situ varies from 1 to 3.8%. Apparently IUCD failure is often due to abnormalities of the uterine cavity, or to a disproportion between the size of the uterine cavity and the size of the IUCD, or the IUCD is incorrectly positioned in the uterus
- A patient will conceive if the IUCD is not in the correct position as expected because then it will not be able to prevent embryo implantation as shown above Experts say that 48 to 56% of patients pregnant with an IUCD in situ will spontaneously abort, that risk of early delivery is 10%, and that the risk of ectopic pregnancy is about 3.4%

The Faculty of Sexual and Reproductive Healthcare of the RCOG published guidance on intrauterine contraception in 2007. This says as follows:
Most pregnancies in patients using intrauterine contraception will be intrauterine but an ectopic pregnancy must be excluded. Patients who become pregnant with an intrauterine contraception in situ should be informed of the increased risks of second-trimester miscarriage, preterm delivery and infection if the intrauterine device is left in situ. Removal would reduce adverse outcomes but is associated with a small risk of miscarriage. If the threads are visible, or can easily be retrieved from the endocervical canal, the intrauterine contraceptive should be removed up to 12 weeks' gestation.
IUCDs are typically removed under ultrasound guidance to lessen the risks of infection, miscarriage, and premature delivery, which can occur if the IUCD is left in place.

3.29
This patient was referred for a scan with a history of positive pregnancy test result with a known IUCD in situ.

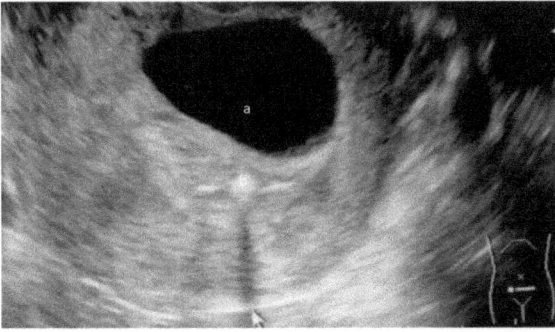
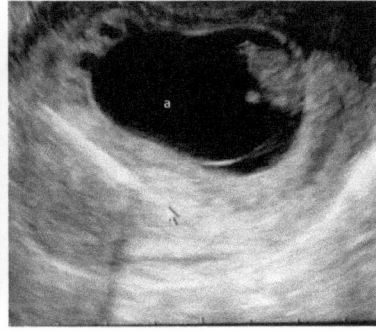

3.29a

a- intrauterine gestational sac

3.29b

c-Copper T IUCD

b- transverse view of Copper T IUCD

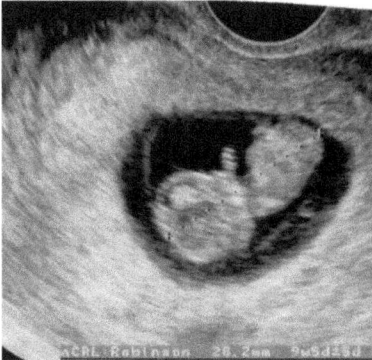
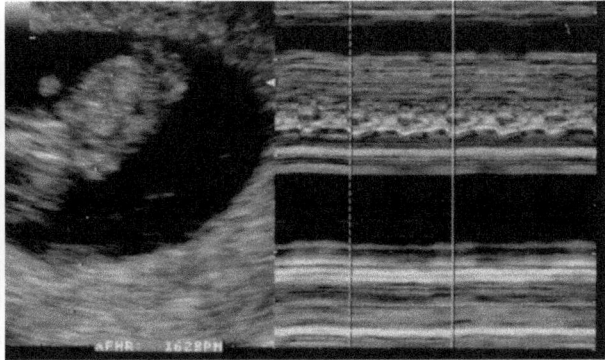

3.29c   **3.29d**

Ultrasound findings: An IUGS, YS and embryonic pole. (3.29a-c) EHR = 162bpm (3.29d) CRL = 28.2mm = 9+5/40(3.29c). Inferior to the GS is a Copper T IUCD (3.29a–b).

Impression: Intrauterine pregnancy with an IUCD in situ.

Pregnancy of unknown location (PUL)

This a condition where there is no sign of either an intra or extrauterine pregnancy or retained products of conception on trans-vaginal ultrasound, despite a positive pregnancy test. Follow-up ultrasound examinations will have to be booked in line with departmental protocol until the ultrasound examination can identify any of the following:

- An ongoing intrauterine pregnancy
- Ectopic pregnancy

- Complete miscarriage or
- Failing PUL – by blood test result

Ultrasound findings will have to be interpreted in line with the clinical assessment of the patient and blood tests (β-hCG) until a diagnosis is reached

Assaults and domestic violence

A pregnant patient may be referred for a scan following assault or domestic violence. The examination is performed as normal. All measurements, embryo or fetal anatomy or any unusual findings should be documented pictorially and in writing, in line with hospital policy, just in case there is legal need for this information at a later date.

Pregnancies following accidents and bad falls

Sometimes a pregnant patient can be referred for a scan having been involved in a road traffic accident or experienced a bad fall. When such a patient with or without her husband or partner presents for a scan, she may be frightened, shaken, fearful, and tearful. The patient may point to a particular place in her abdomen or pelvis as her area(s) of pain or concern.

The sonographer in addition to performing the examination professionally should endeavour to check the areas that the patient highlights. These patients may need extra kindness and attention. The examination is performed as normal. All measurements, embryo or fetal anatomy or any unusual findings should be documented pictorially and in writing in line with the hospital protocol.

Maternal anxiety

Pregnant patients can sometimes get referred for a scan especially in the first trimester because of maternal anxiety, which can be as a result of factors including the following:

> Previous missed abortion
> ? not feeling pregnant again
> Unexplainable vaginal bleeding
> Previous bad obstetric history
> After a fall

Once the sonographer has established the location of the pregnancy and confirmed that there are embryonic or fetal hearbeats and movements, it is good practice that the couple be informed before the sonographer continues the examination.

Patients with known severe haemophilia

Haemophilia is passed to a child by one or both of their parents. Haemophilia A and B is inherited as an X-linked recessive bleeding disorder. Therefore, maternal carriers have a 50% chance of delivering an affected male infant. When the mother is a known haemophiliac (A or B carrier) and with an ongoing pregnancy, it is important that fetal sexing is performed as part of the antenatal care as this will affect her pregnancy management. Fetal sexing is undertaken either by maternal blood sampling at around 10 weeks' gestation or by an ultrasound scan between 18 and 20 weeks. For the maternal blood sampling to be carried out at the appropriate GA, an ultrasound dating scan is mandatory hence such a patient would be referred for a dating scan irrespective of her LMP. If the maternal blood screening test shows that the fetus is a male, then diagnostic tests can be arranged to confirm whether the baby would definitely have the disease or not, and the pregnancy would then be monitored as per the national guidelines.

3.30

This patient was referred for a dating scan with a history of severe haemophilia. LMP – Unsure. Both ovaries (not shown here) appear sonographically normal.

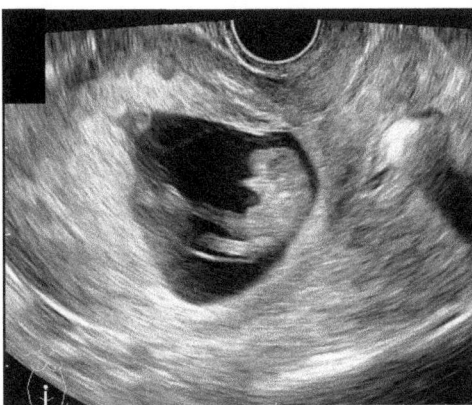

3.30a

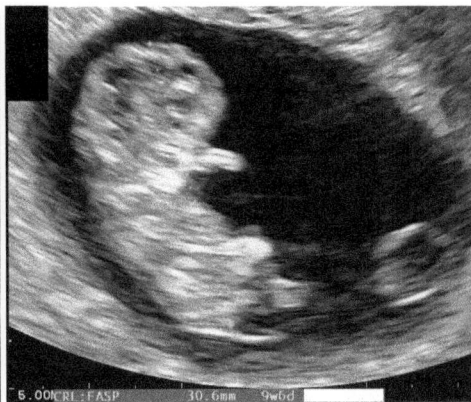

3.30b

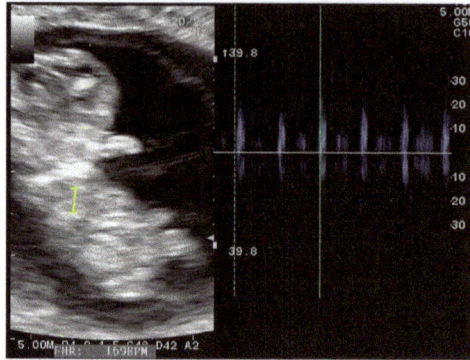

3.30c

Ultrasound findings: Single intrauterine pregnancy.
CRL = 30.6 = 9+6/40 (3.30b). EHR = 169bpm (3.30c).

Impression: Single ongoing intrauterine pregnancy.

Abdominal or pelvic pain and bleeding

As much as possible, the patient should be asked to describe the location and nature of her abdominal pain. She should be asked to use one of her fingers to pinpoint the location of the pain. In addition to assessing the pregnancy, the sonographer should endeavour to carefully scan the area to find the source of the pain in the area of intense pain and the findings should be documented. It is not unusual not to be able to identify GIT problems if or when that is the cause of the pain. Ultrasound identifiable causes of pain in pregnancy include the following:

- Fibroids
- Ectopic pregnancy
- Ongoing miscarriage or abortion
- Ovarian cysts ± ovarian torsion
- Normal fetal parts, e.g. elbow, feet (uncommon in 1st trimester)
- Fetus ignorantly kicking a maternal fibroid or resting his/her feet or head on it
- Lots of bowel gas – GIT problems may not be excluded
- Appendicitis – this pain is always in the patient's right iliac fossa (RIF).

Finding a normal right ovary in a patient with RIF pain should raise the suspicion of appendicitis and the patient should be referred to the main ultrasound department for further ultrasound examination especially if the sonographer in the EPAGU is not trained to examine the appendix or if the appropriate ultrasound probe is not available in EPAGU.

3.31

This patient was referred for a scan due to sudden abdominal pains that day. GA by LMP = 6+1. Left ovary was not visualised.

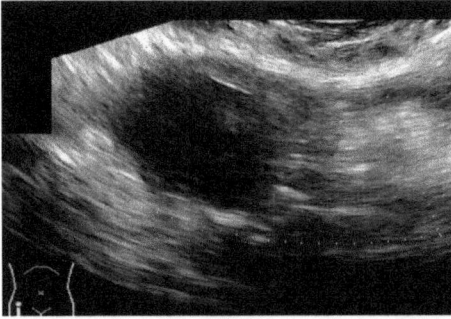 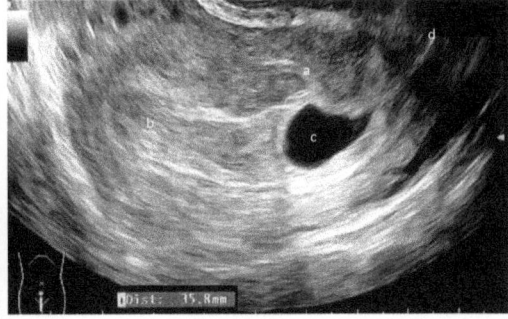

3.31a	**3.31b**

a-previous C/S scar, b- endometrium, c-gestational sac, d-cervical canal

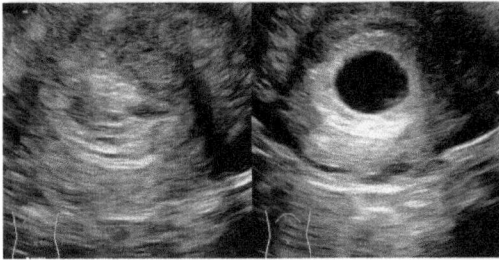 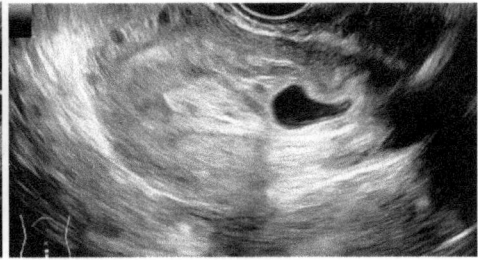

3.31c	**3.31d**

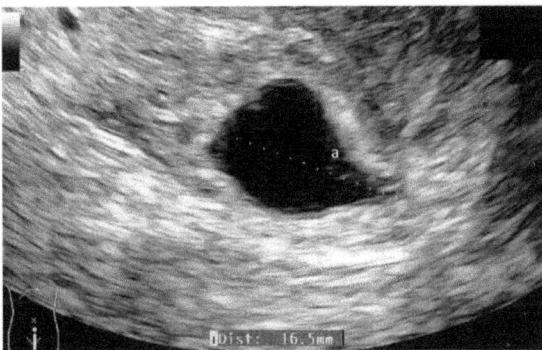

3.31e a-yolk sac

Ultrasound findings: Just inferior to a previous c/s scar is a slightly irregular in outline gestational sac measuring approx.16.5mm in diameter. There is a yolk sac but no fetal pole (3.31e). There is a simple cyst in the right ovary (3.31a). The left ovary was not visualised.

Impression: IUGS inferior to the c/s scar

 ? impending miscarriage

Normal early cervical pregnancy

This patient was rescheduled for another scan 7 days later.

Follow-up showed a complete miscarriage.

3.32

This patient was referred with a history of pelvic pain. The patient was tender over the area adjacent to the gestational sac as shown below.

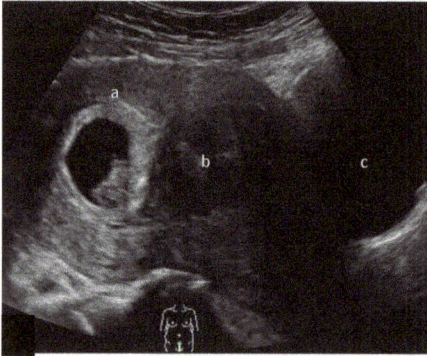 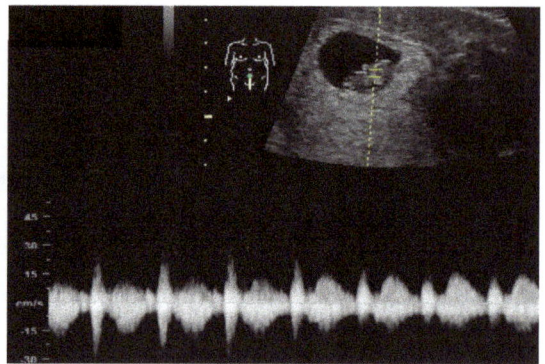

3.32a **3.32b**

a- IUGS, b-fibroid, c- maternal urinary bladder

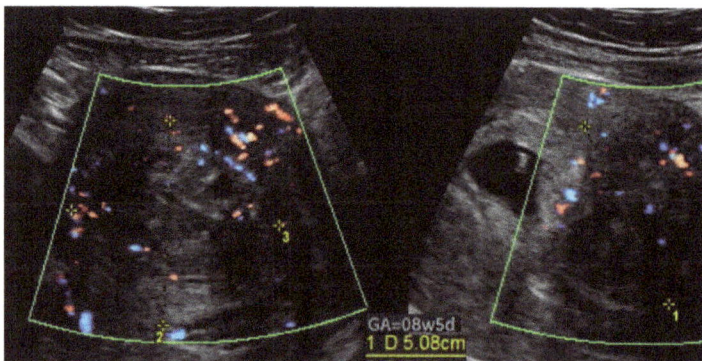

3.32c

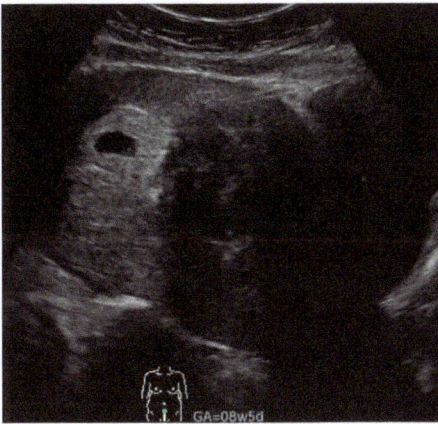

3.32d

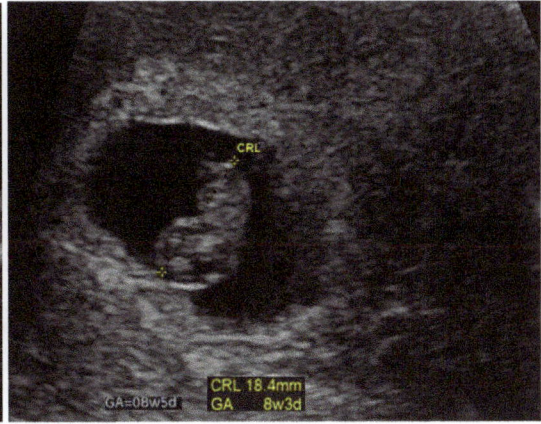

3.32e

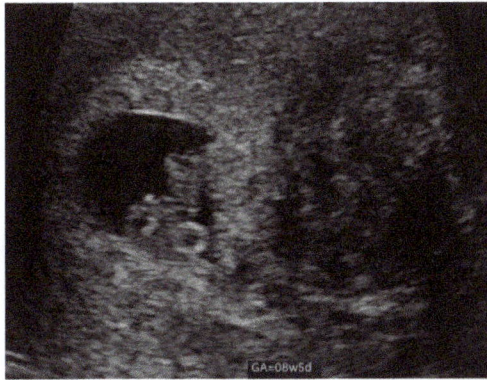

3.32f

Ultrasound findings: There is an intrauterine gestational sac, yolk sac, embryonic pole (3.32a, e–f) and EHB (3.32b). CRL = 18.4mm = 8+3/40. There is also an approx. 51 × 53 × 55mm intramural anterior cervical fibroid with possible cystic component in the centre (3.32a, c–e). This area corresponds to the area of the patient's pain. ?degenerating fibroid (in 3.32a & d) (red degeneration).

Impression: Intrauterine pregnancy. Anterior possible red degenerating cervical fibroid.

* It is believed that red or carneous degeneration is due to haemorrhagic infarction, which can occur particularly during pregnancy, and may present with acute abdominal pain.

Fibroids in pregnancy

What do fibroids in pregnancy mean and what documentation is needed when they are reported in a scan?

A fibroid is a non-cancerous tumour that grows from the uterine muscle and could be located within the endometrial cavity or anywhere in the myometrium or outside the womb. Fibroids may be connected with stalks and these are known as pedunculated fibroids.

Once a fibroid is identified, there is need for its documentation as follows:

- Location of the fibroid(s), size and how many. Documenting the size of a fibroid helps to monitor if it grows or not during the pregnancy
- Will it affect or impede normal delivery?
  A fibroid can become painful in pregnancy because it is degenerating (undergoing 'red degeneration'), torsion if pedunculated or impaction or because the baby is lying on the intramural or subserosal fibroid or kicking it innocently
- It is estimated that approximately 10% to 30% of patients with fibroids develop complications during pregnancy
- In early pregnancy, spontaneous miscarriage rates are quoted as greatly increased in pregnant patients with fibroids compared with those without fibroids
- It has been said that bleeding is significantly more common if the placenta implants close to the fibroid. In late pregnancy, such complications include preterm labour, placental abruption, placenta praevia, and fetal anomalies
- Pain is the most common complication of fibroids during pregnancy

Abnormal bleeding and +ve pregnancy tests until 18/40

This is one of the commonest reasons for patients needing a scan especially in the first trimester of pregnancy. Any form of vaginal bleeding can be very frightening and a patient may attend the unit with much fear. Bleeding may be painless or painful with or without abdominal or pelvic pain. Bleeding may comprise that which a patient sees after wiping herself in the toilet or a few spots of blood on the knickers, or light bleeding or heavy bleeding. It may be unprovoked bleeding or occur after a walk or exercise, or after carrying some shopping, or lifting or moving the furniture, or even after making love. These patients are often very anxious; often they think they have just lost their babies. It is good practice, once the pregnancy is confirmed to be intrauterine and the fetal heart beat is seen, for the sonographer to inform the patient and show her this on the TV monitor before he proceeds to check the embryonic or fetal anatomy, adnexa and complete the scan in line with the protocol. Ultrasound evidence or cause of the bleeding should be sought for and documented. Sometimes no ultrasound features can be seen to confirm the bleed. Ultrasound identifiable causes for vaginal bleeding include the following:

- Missed abortion or missed miscarriage
- Molar pregnancy
- Implantational bleed
- Subchorionic haematoma
- Ongoing or incomplete miscarriage
- Ectopic pregnancy – many times with abdominal or pelvic pain
- Decidual reaction in the non-pregnant horn of a bicornuate uterus or uterus didelphys

When the bleeding is associated with pain, the patient should pinpoint the location of the pain and the sonographer should endeavour to carefully scan the area to find the source or cause of the pain.

- It is believed that 1 in 4 to 1 in 5 of pregnant patients will experience some kind of bleeding especially in the first trimester of their pregnancy. However, more than half of these patients who bleed in the first trimester go on to have a perfectly healthy pregnancy
- It is common not to find any ultrasound evidence of bleeding in patients who have vaginal bleeding after sexual intercourse, otherwise known as post-coital bleeding
- Trauma or tears to the vaginal wall or some infections can also cause bleeding in pregnancy in which case there may be no obvious ultrasound evidence for the bleeding

3.33

This was a natural conception and the patient was referred because of spotting in pregnancy.

3.33a   3.33b

3.33c   3.33d

a-There is a tiny hypoechoic area just above the lambda sign, this is likely to be a small implantational bleed

Ultrasound findings: Dizygotic diamniotic twins. Note the lambda sign (3.33a & d). EHB seen in both twins 162bpm and 174bpm (3.33c–d). CRL = 21.2mm and 22.7mm (3.33b). Note the difference in the EHB and CRLs. There is a tiny hypoechoic area just above the lambda sign, note the arrows in (3.33a & d). This is likely to be a small implantational bleed.

Impression: Dizygotic, diamniotic twins.

Dizygotic twins

Develop from two ova

Begin as two separate zygotes

Do not have to be the same sex

Genetically no more identical than two siblings from the same parents

The greater CRL is used in dating a twin or multiple pregnancy. It is important that the chorionicity of a twin pregnancy is established as early as possible in the pregnancy as it has pregnancy-related implications and on how the pregnancy is followed up or monitored

Confirming the chorionicity is a lot easier in the late first trimester as opposed to waiting till the second trimester

It is not unusual in multiple pregnancy

Not to be able to get the embryos or fetuses lying in the same direction

Not to be able to see them together at the same time on the screen

That the CRL and FHB may not be exactly the same

It is important for the sonographer who discovers the multiple pregnancy first to identify the type of pregnancy. For instance, is it DC/DA, MC/MA, MC/DA? Their presentations in relation to the maternal cervix or abdomen (when the presentation becomes obvious not in early pregnancy). The presenting twin is always called twin 1. For example:

Twin 1 is breech and on the maternal left;

Twin 2 is cephalic and on the maternal right.

Once this presentation has been established, subsequent ultrasound reports must always reflect their position(s) in the maternal pelvis or abdomen

3.34

This patient was referred for a scan with a history of spotting for 1/7.

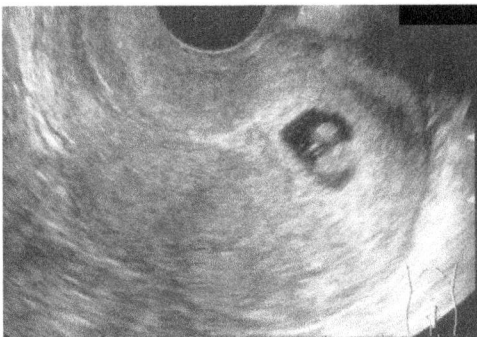 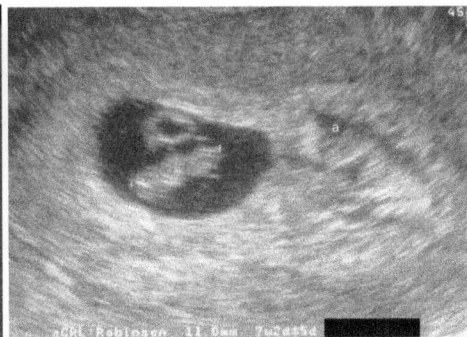

3.34a   **3.35b**

a. (3.34a & 3.34d arrows)

a-an echo poor area to the right of the gestational sac, this is probably an implantational bleed

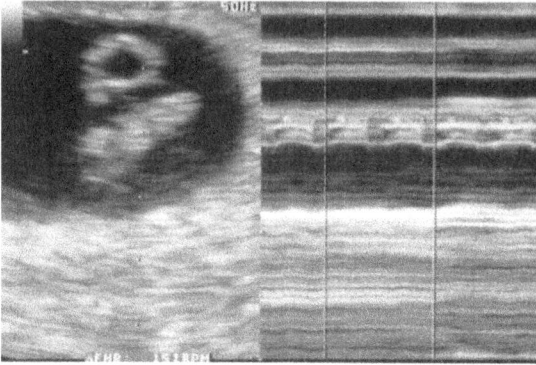
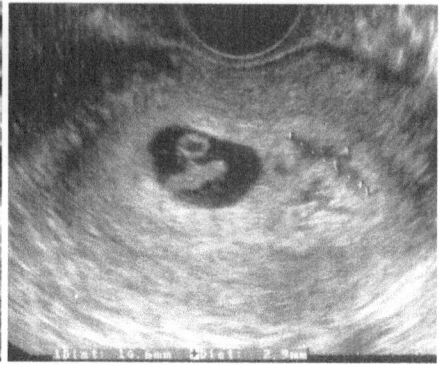

| 3.34c | 3.34d |

Ultrasound findings: Retroverted uterus (3.34a) with a single intrauterine gestational sac, yolk sac, embryonic pole (3.34a–b). CRL = 11mm = 7+2/40 (3.34b). EHB (3.34c). There is an echo poor area to the left of the gestational sac (3.34d). This is probably an implantational bleed (3.34b & 3.34d).

Impression: Threatened abortion or miscarriage

*There is no clinical justification for performing weekly scans just for maternal reassurance.

Implantional bleeds

These bleeds occur secondary to the blastocyst trying to implant in the endometrium and leaving some blood behind. Sometimes these small bleeds are reabsorbed and patients may complain of light to dark or brownish-pink discharge. Patients have described this form of bleeding as vaginal discharge or blood that is not like the menstrual period.

It is important to confirm or exclude an intrauterine gestational sac (IUGS), yolk sac (YS), embryonic or fetal pole (EP or FP), embryonic or fetal heart beats (EHB or FHB). Significant areas of bleeding should be measured and documented as they may have an effect on the pregnancy. In addition, further scans may be needed to assess this form of bleeding.

3.35

This patient was referred with a history of vaginal bleeding.

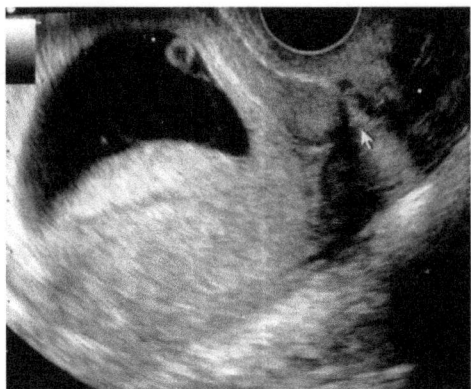 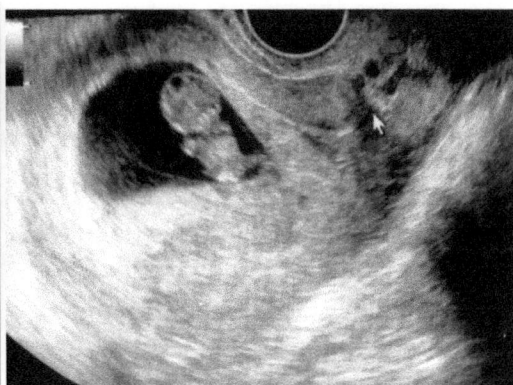

3.35a   **3.35b**

Arrow shows the previous c/s scar in 3.35a & 3.35b.

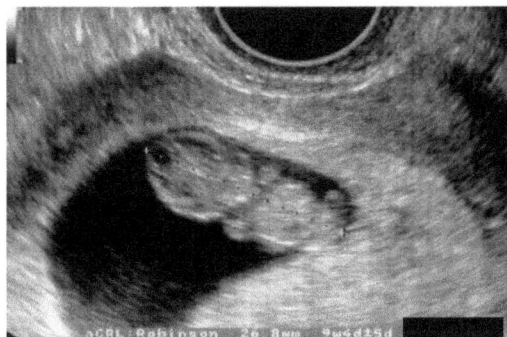 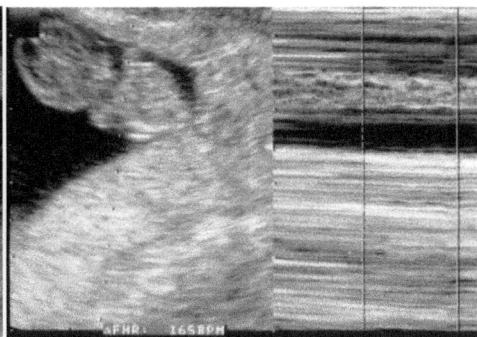

3.35c   **3.35d**

Ultrasound findings: Single intrauterine gestational sac, yolk sac, embryo (3.35a–b), EHB is seen. EHR = 165bpm (3.35d). CRL = 26.8mm = 9+4/40 (3.35c). Previous c/s scar is noted. A small implantation bleed cannot be excluded.

Impression: Singleton intrauterine gestation with EHB. This is an example of threatened abortion or miscarriage.

3.36

This patient was referred at 6/40 with a history of bleeding.

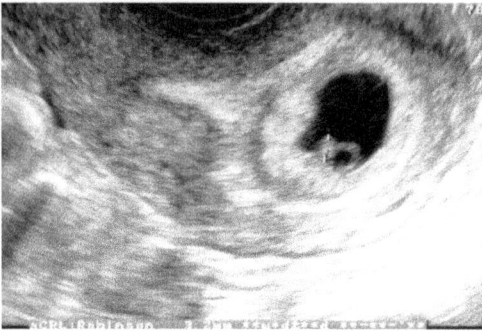

3.36a

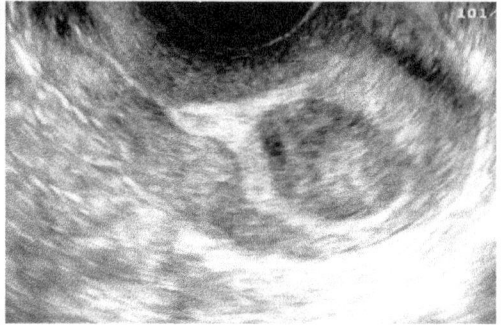

3.36b

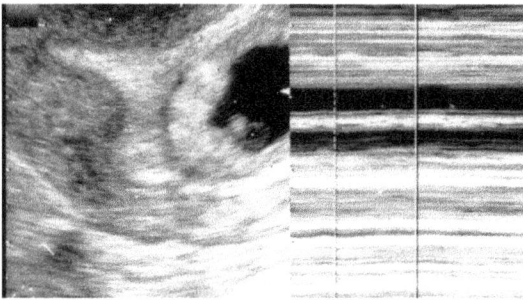

3.36c

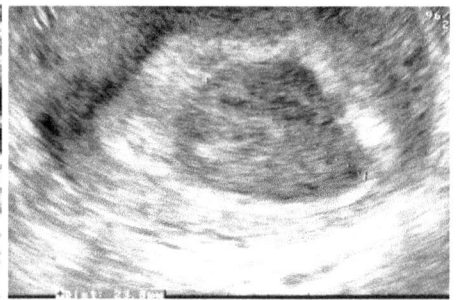

3.36d

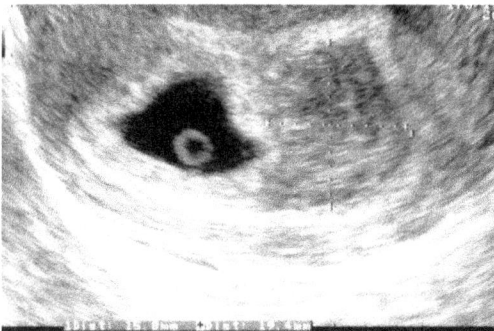

3.36e

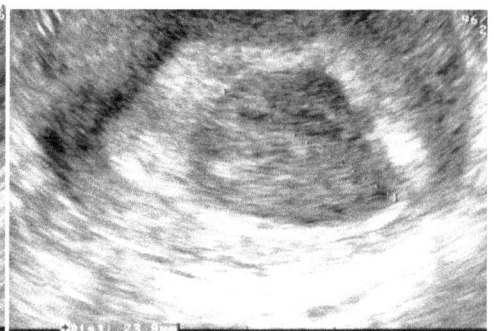

3.36f

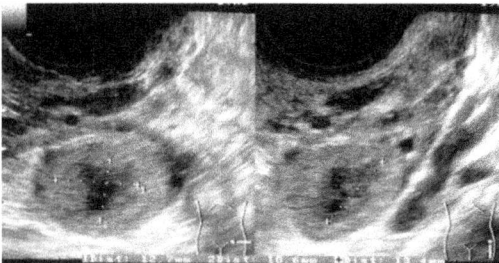

3.36g

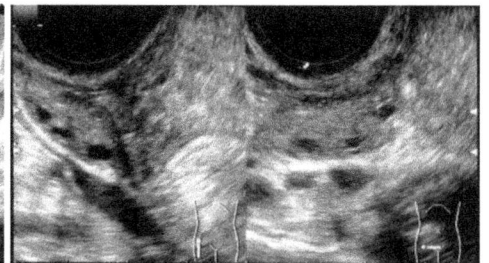

3.36h

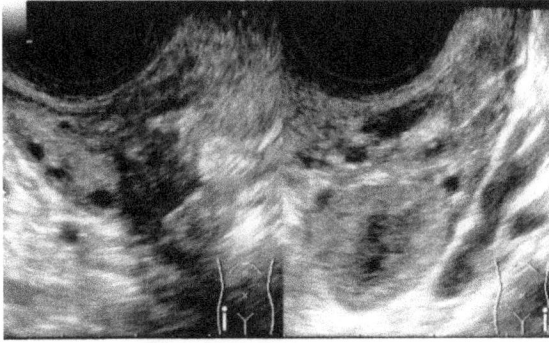

3.36i

Ultrasound findings: Bicornuate retroverted uterus (3.36a–b & e). There is an intrauterine gestation sac in the right horn. Single fetus, YS, EP and EHB (3.36a, c & e). CRL = 3.2mm (3.36a). The left horn is filled with hypoechoic materials measuring approx. 16 × 19 × 24mm (3.36 b, d–f). There is an approx. 10 × 13 × 13mm corpus luteum in the left ovary (3.36g). The right ovary appears normal (measurements are not included 3.36h and first half of i).

Impression: Bicornuate uterus. The pregnancy is in the right horn. There is a decidual reaction in the left horn and that is probably the cause of the bleeding. Experts believe that bicornuate uterus can cause preterm labour and possible cervical insufficiency but not in the first trimester of pregnancy.

Both cervical insufficiency and preterm delivery can cause a miscarriage or baby loss at birth where and when the baby is born prematurely.

3.37
This patient was referred with a history of vaginal bleeding at 8/40.

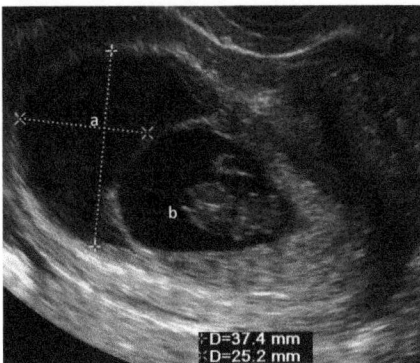

3.37a

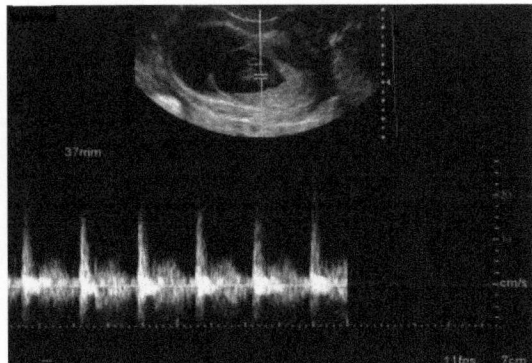

3.37b

a-Superior and to the right of the gestational sac is an approx. 37 × 25 × 20.5mm low-level echoed cystic area (3.38 a & c). This is probably a subchorionic haematoma or haemorrhage. b- gestational sac,

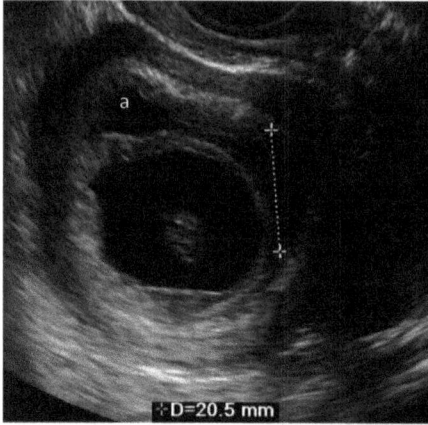 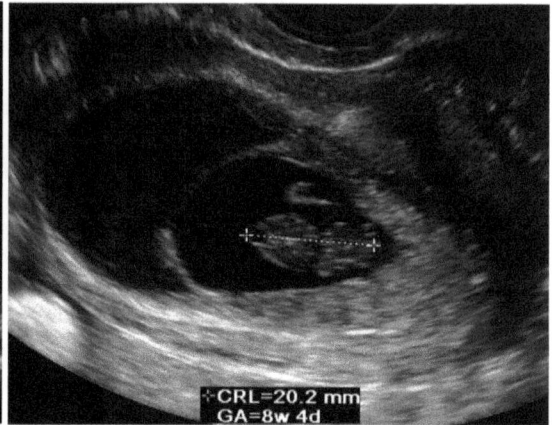

3.37c   **3.37d**

a- superior and to the right of the gestational sac is an approx. 37 × 25 × 20.5mm low-level echoed cystic area (3.38 a & c). This is probably a subchorionic haematoma or hemorrhage.

Ultrasound findings: An intrauterine gestational sac, embryonic pole and EHB (3.37a – b). CRL = 20.2mm = 8+4/40 (3.37d). To the right of the gestational sac is an approx. 37 × 25 × 20.5mm low-level echoed cystic area (3.37a & c). This is probably a subchorionic haematoma or hemorrhage.

Differential diagnoses will include a co-existing empty gestational sac.

Impression: An ongoing IUP with some subchorionic haematoma or hemorrhage. Subchorionic haemorrhage or haematomas have been linked to an increased risk of miscarriage, stillbirth, placental abruption and preterm labour. It is believed that for patients with a subchorionic haematoma that issonographically identified, fetal outcome is dependent on the size of the haematoma, maternal age, and gestational age

Miscarriage rates are said to increase with maternal age. The size of the haematoma is believed may have an impact on the pregnancy outcome. It is beleived that the larger the haematoma the more likely that it may lead to complications, such as stripping the placenta away from the uterus, compressing the gestational sac and leading to premature rupture of the membranes (PROM) with consequent spontaneous abortion

Follow-up: Haematoma gradually reduced in size but was still seen at the NT scan some weeks later

3.38

This patient was referred with a history of spotting in early pregnancy. Both ovaries (not shown here) appeared sonographically normal. EHB × 2 were seen.

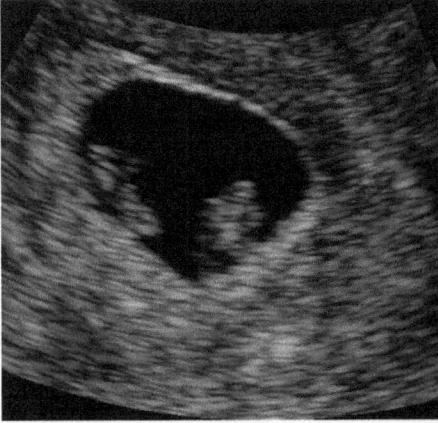

3.38a

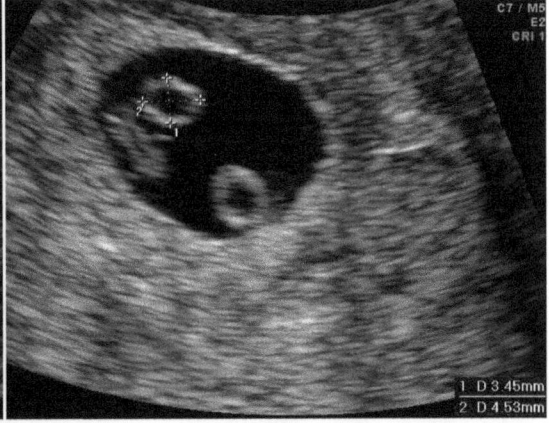

3.38b

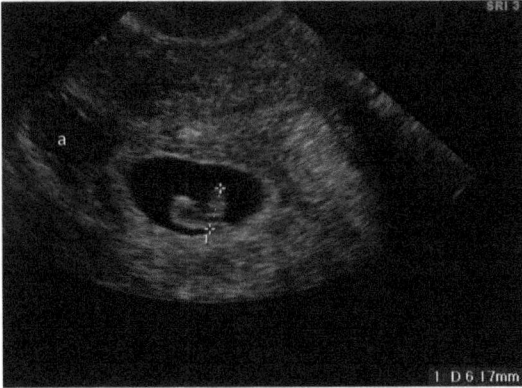

3.38c

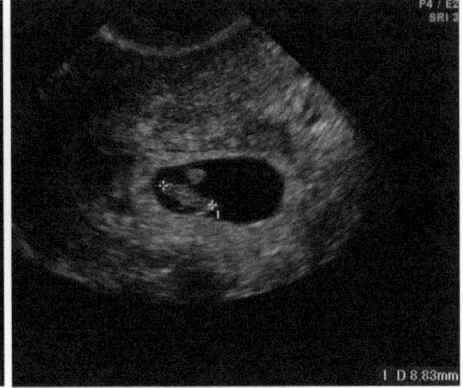

3.89d

a-small area, a possible bleed, adjacent and slightly superior and to the right of the gestational sac

Ultrasound findings: Single intrauterine gestational sac, two YS, two EPS. (3.38a–

b) CRL = 8.3mm, CRL = 6.2 mm (3.38c–d). Usually the pregnancy is dated by the greater CRL.

Impression: Monochorionic (MC) pregnancy.

Note the small area, a possible bleed, to the right of the gestational sac in 3.38c–d. A follow-up should be arranged for 2–3 weeks from then to check if it will be two amniotic sacs or one, i.e. MC/MA or MC/DA

MC twins have the highest mortality (10–40%) of an uncomplicated twin pregnancy. They are prone to an increased incidence of congenital anomalies, cord entanglement, prematurity and twin-to-twin transfusion syndrome (TTTS)

They usually have one placenta

Further scan appointments should be twice the time allocated per singleton pregnancy

Whilst it may be exciting for the sonographer to find a multiple pregnancy, it should be remembered that this might actually be 'social bad news' for the patient as not every patient is excited about the prospects of a multiple pregnancy, especially if she has had other children before the current pregnancy or for her social circumstances.

Maternal cysts in pregnancy – *what do they mean?*

Cysts, discovered during a pregnancy scan, are often an accidental finding (non-symptomatic cysts). On the other hand, in the process of trying to identify the cause of abdominal or pelvic pain a cyst may be found (symptomatic findings).

It is always a good practice to examine the patient's adnexa when performing any obstetric scan. All identified cysts should be measured and documented with the following information:

- Where exactly is the cyst(s), i.e. location?
- Is the ovary seen with or without the cyst?
- Size of the cyst
- Description of the cyst(s) including its margin and wall
- Is the cyst(s) vascular on Doppler or not?
- The type of cyst, e.g. corpus luteum, simple, haemorrhagic, dermoid, complex, suspicious malignant
- Whether the cyst should be monitored in pregnancy or post-pregnancy

Large cysts may cause abdominal or pelvic pain, may be prone to torsion or rupture which are reasons for a patient to visit the emergency department of the hospital.

3.39

This patient was referred because she required a dating scan.

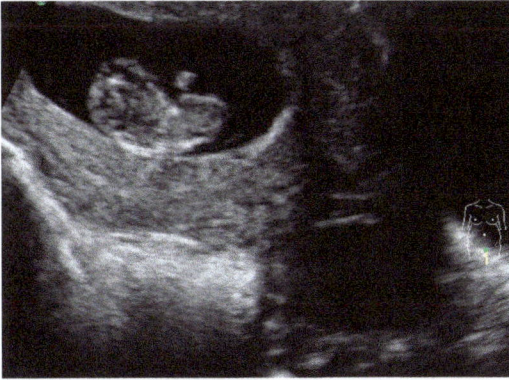

3.39a

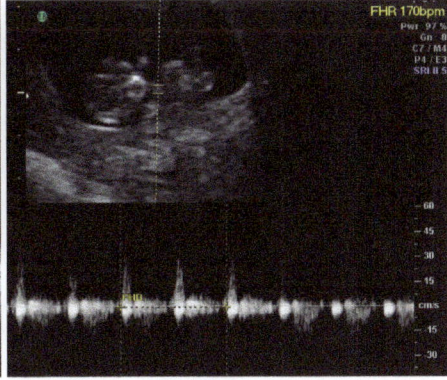

3.39b

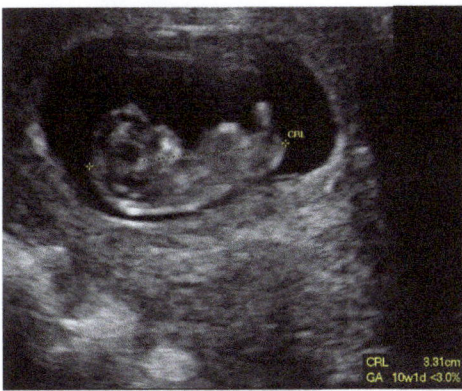

3.39c

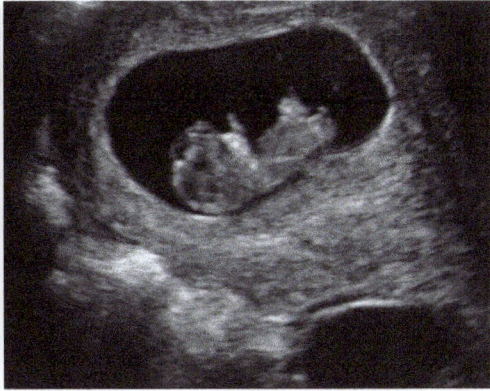

3.39d

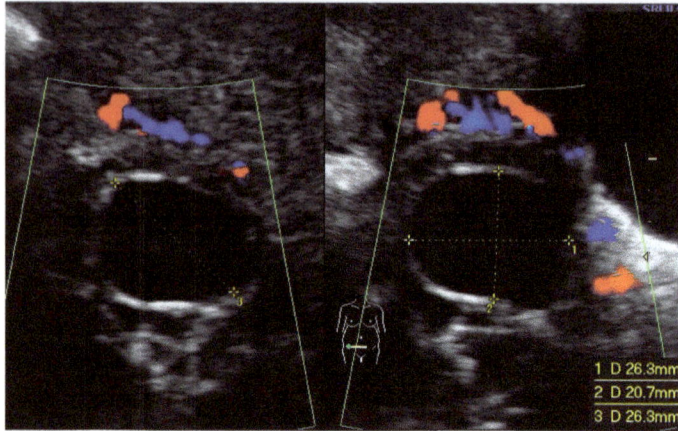

3.39e

Ultrasound findings: Single intrauterine gestation, fetus (3.39a & c) and FHB (3.39b). CRL = 3.31cm = 10+1/40 (3.39c). There is a 26 × 21 × 26mm cyst with an echogenic ring in the right adnexa inferior to the uterus (3.39d–e). It is not a corpus luteal cyst as there is no ultrasound evidence of the 'ring of fire' around it. **Impression:** Single intrauterine gestation, fetus and FHB. Cyst in the right adnexa.

3.40

This patient was referred with a history of LIF pain and a positive pregnancy test.

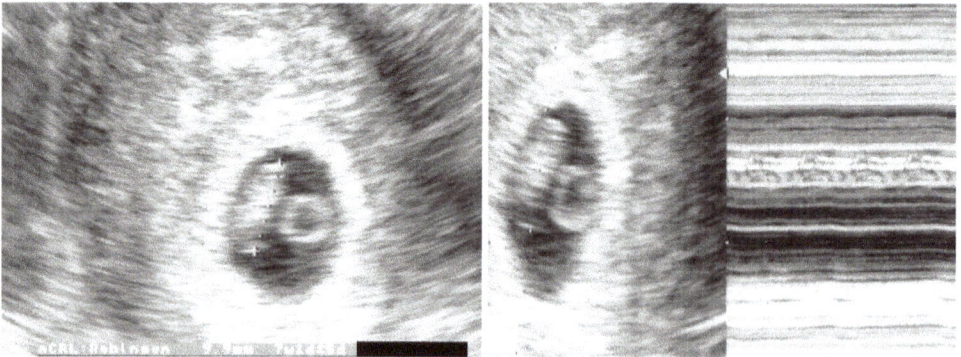

3.40a   **3.40b**

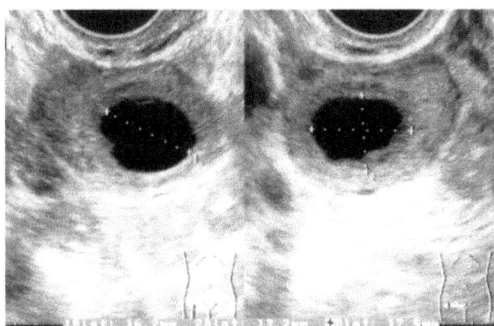

3.40c

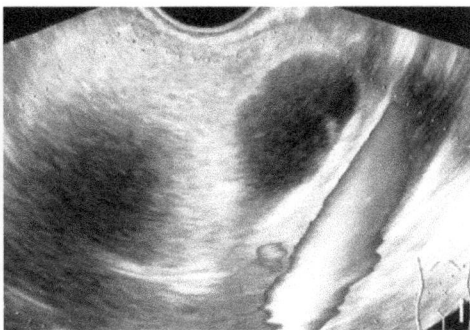

3.40d

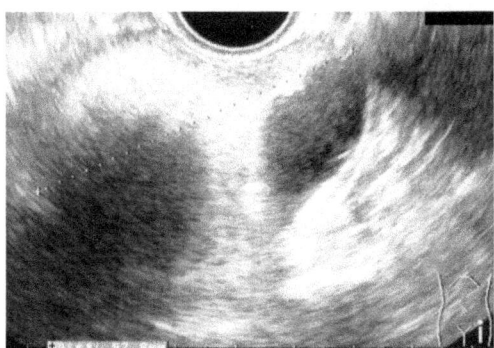

3.40e

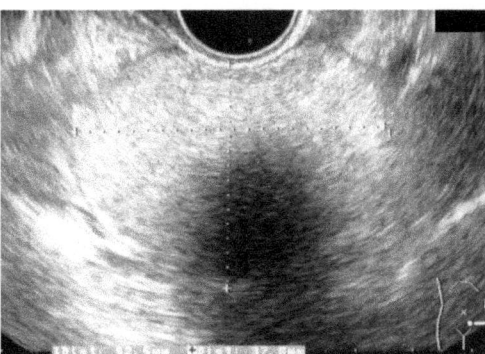

3.40f

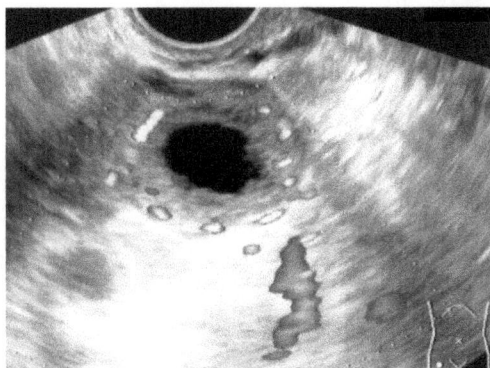

3.40g

Ultrasound findings: An intrauterine gestational sac, YS, embryo and EHB (3.40a–b). CRL = 9.5mm = 7+1/40 (3.40b). There is a corpus luteum in the right ovary (3.40c & g). In the left adnexa is an approx. 58 × 53 × 38mm predominantly hyperechoic avascular structure with two hypoechoic entities in it. The left ovary is not demonstrated separately from this entity. (3.40d–f)

Impression: Single IUP with EHB. Corpus luteum in the right ovary. Dermoid cyst in the left ovary.

Suggest a follow-up scan in 2–3 weeks from that day to confirm or refute if the pregnancy is ongoing or otherwise and probably date the pregnancy accurately.

3.41

This patient was referred because of bleeding in pregnancy. The ultrasound findings are shown below. FHB and movements were seen (not shown here).

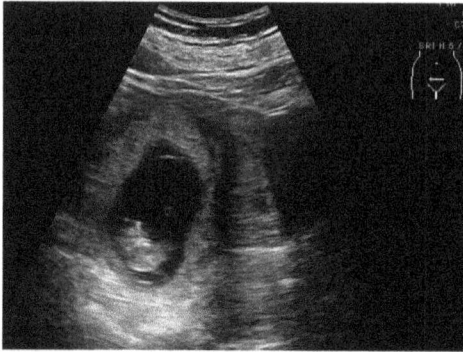

3.41a

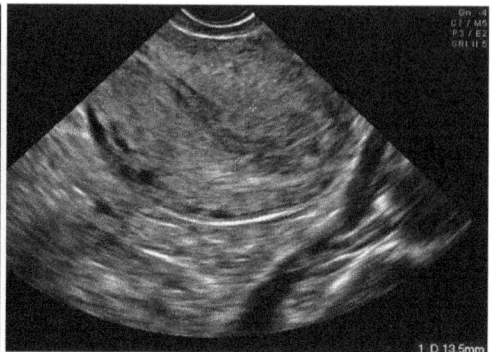

3.41b

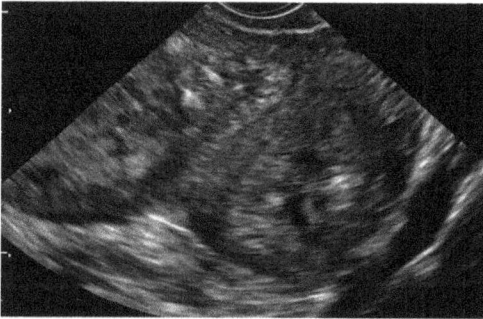

3.41c

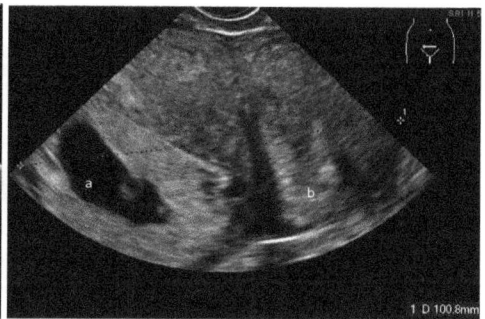

3.41d

3.41d. Uterus didelphys a- an intrauterine gestational sac in the right horn, b- endometrial thickening in the left horn which probably is the cause of the vaginal bleeding for this patient.

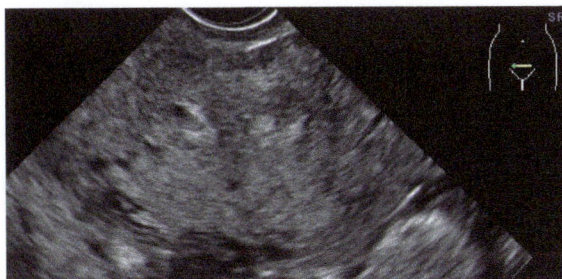 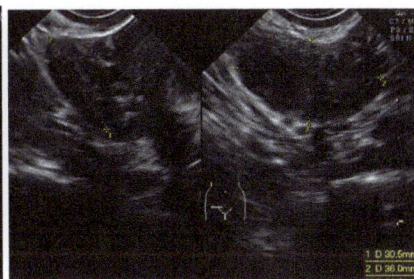

3.41e   **3.41f**

Note the two cervices above.

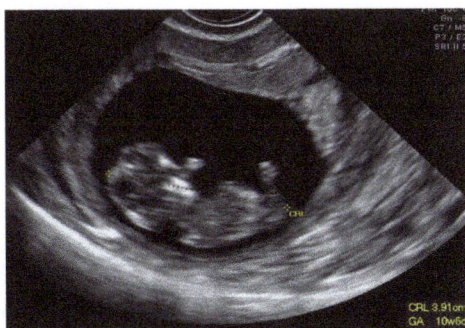

3.41g

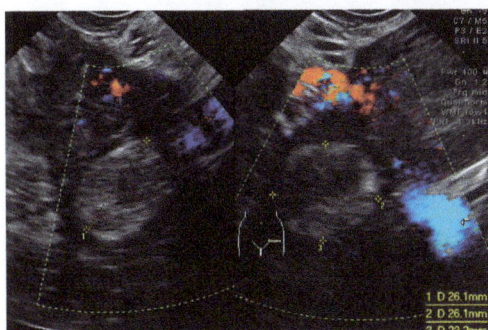 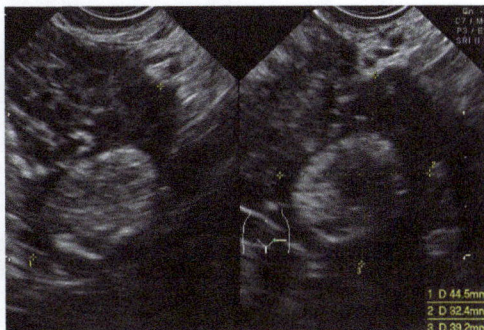

3.41h   **3.41i**

Ultrasound findings: Uterus didelphys (3.41a, c & e) with an intrauterine gestational sac. Fetus, in the right horn (3.41a, d & g). CRL = 39.1mm= 10+6/40 (3.41g). There is endometrial thickening in the left horn 3.41b–d (decidual reaction) which probably is the cause of the vaginal bleeding for this patient. The left ovary measures 45 × 39 × 32mm and in it is an approx. 26 × 23 × 26mm smooth in outline avascular echogenic area (3.41h–i). The right ovary measures 31 × 36 × 20mm (3.41f).

Impression: Uterus didelphys with the pregnancy in the right horn. The right ovary appears sonographically normal. Ultrasound appearance of the left ovary is suggestive of a dermoid cyst. Uterine differentials – Bicornuate uterus.

With uterus didelphys there will be two distinct normal-sized uterine cavities and two cervices

Uterus didelphys is associated with a high incidence of unilateral renal agenesis

Unlike some other uterine abnormalities, experts believe that uterus didelphys does not significantly affect the obstetric outcome

Incidence rate of uterus didelphys is estimated or quoted as I in 3000 patients

3.42

This patient was referred with a history of anxiety and pvb. Natural conception. GA by LMP = 5+4/40.

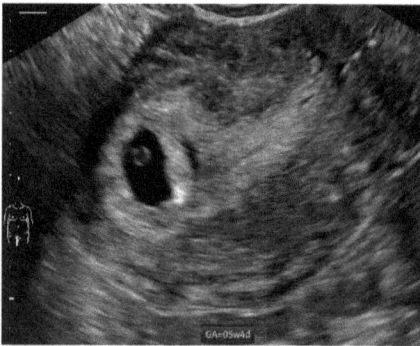

3.42a

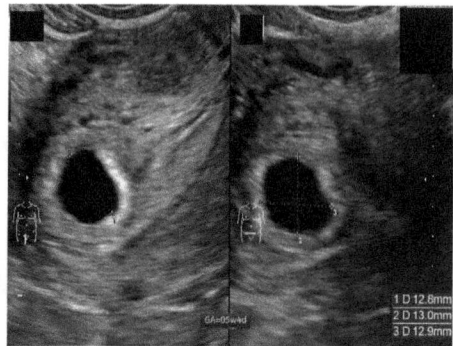

3.42b (13 x 13 x 13mm)

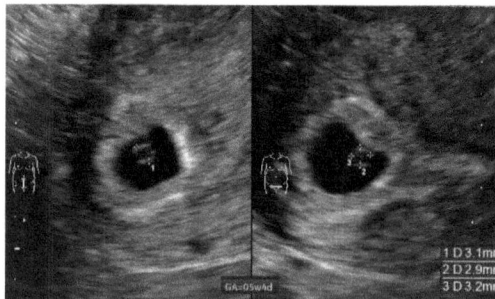

3.42c (3 x 3 x 3mm)

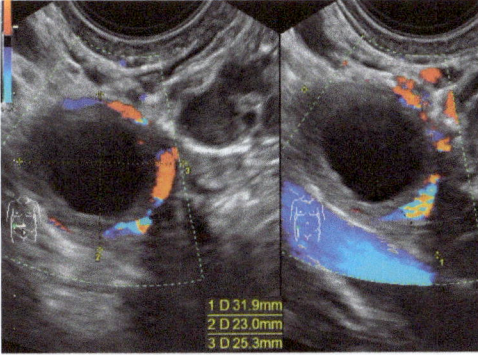

3.42d (32 x 23 x 25mm)

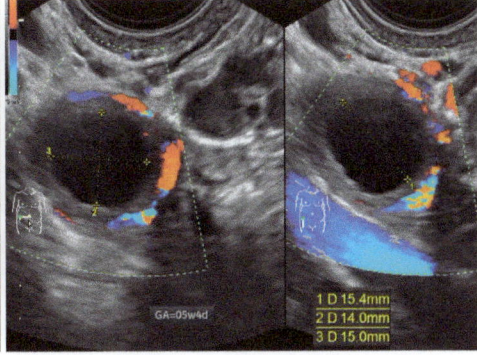

3.42e (15 x 14 x 15mm)

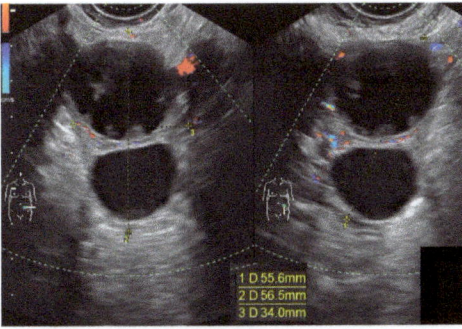

3.42f

(56 x 56 x 34mm)

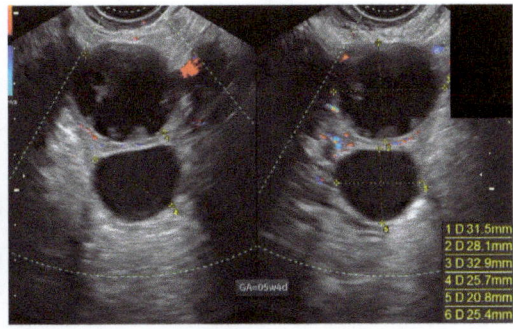

3.42g

(32 x 28 x 33mm, 26 x 21 x 25mm)

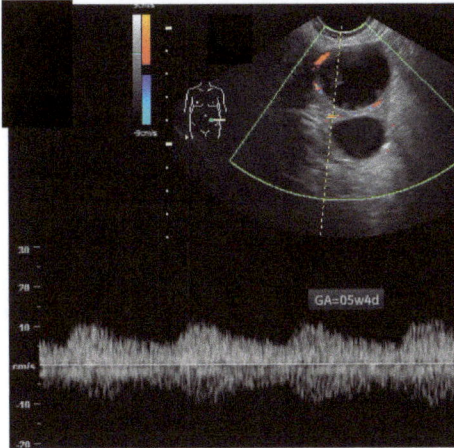

3.42h

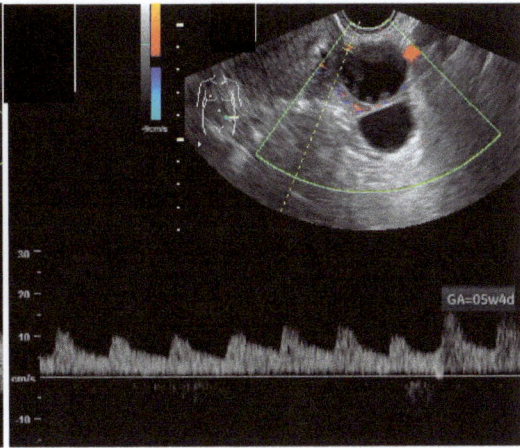

3.42i

Ultrasound report: An IUGS measuring 13 x 13 x 13mm with a YS measuring 3 x 3 x 3mm. No EP is demonstrated. No obvious ultrasound evidence or cause for pvb is demonstrated. The right ovary is measuring 32 x 23 x 25mm (9.6mls) and in it is a 15 x 14 x 15mm corpus luteum. The left ovary is measuring 56 x 56 x 34mm (55.8mls) and in it are two septated cystic areas measuring 32 x 28 x 33mm and 26 x 21 x 25mm. The larger one of the cysts is vascular on Colour flow Dopplers and has tiny scattered echogenic areas.

Impression: An early pregnancy. Normal right ovary. Left ovarian pathology cannot be excluded and this will require appropriate follow up

Nausea and or vomiting or hyperemesis gravidarum

Nausea and vomiting occurs in 50–90% of pregnancies. Hyperemesis gravidarum is a condition that affects less than 0.5% of pregnant patients and it is the most severe form of nausea and vomiting. It is believed that pregnancy-related nausea and vomiting often starts by 9–10/40 reaching its peak at 11–13/40, with most resolving by 12–14 weeks' gestation. It is claimed that 1% of cases may be symptomatic even past 20–22/40. Ultrasound examinations of such patients are carried out in order to:

Confirm if it is a singleton or multiple pregnancy
Date the pregnancy
Exclude or confirm hydatidiform mole
Patients who are prone to this condition include:

- Those who have had the condition before

- First pregnancies

- Patients who are undergoing extreme psychological stress

- Patients with electrolyte imbalances or vitamin B deficiencies

- Patients who have Helicobacter pylori infection

3.43
This patient was referred because of hyperemesis. Both ovaries appeared sonographically normal.

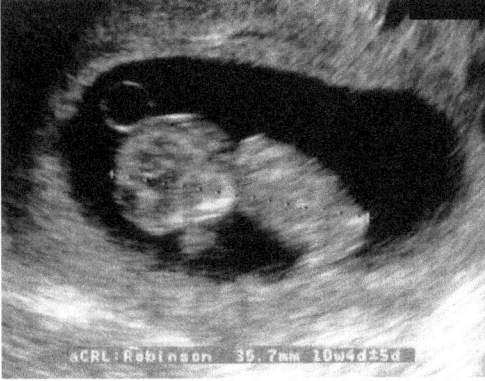 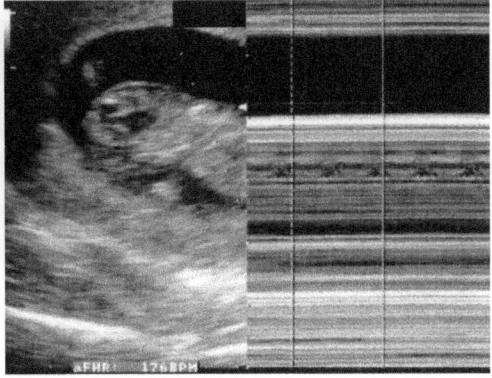

3.43a   **3.43b**

Ultrasound findings: Single IUP (3.46a). Fetal pole with a FHB of 174 bpm
(3.43b). CRL = 35.7mm = 10+4/40 (3.43b)

Impression: Ongoing singleton IUP.

3.44

This patient was referred because of hyperemesis post IVF conception. FET
x 2. GA by IVF treatment was 7+3/40. Ist scan in the pregnancy. Both ovaries
not shown here were enlarged measuring over 100mls each and with multiple
corpus luteal cysts.

Ultrasound findings:

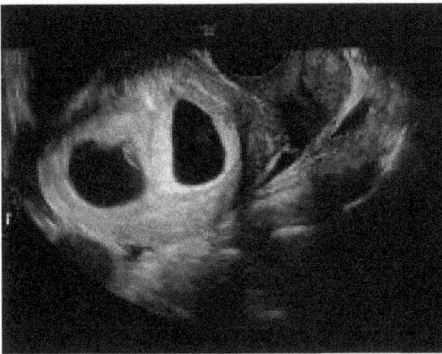 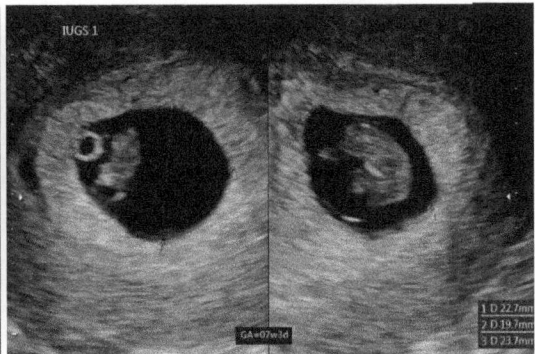

3.44a   **3.44b**

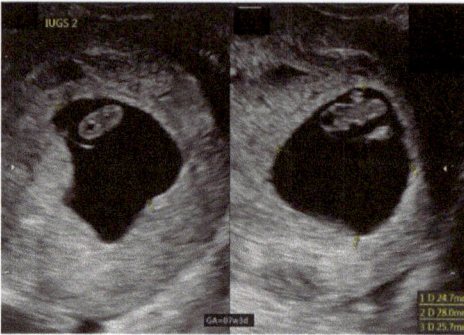

3.44c

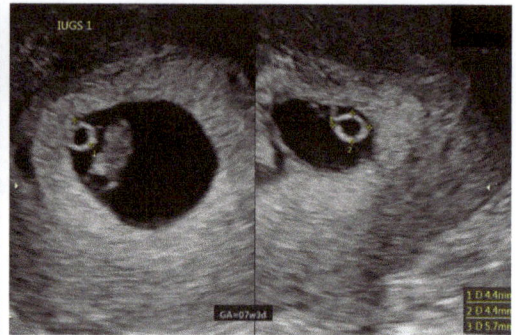

3.44d

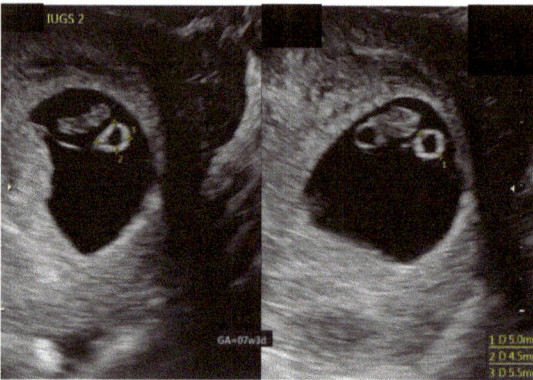

3.44e

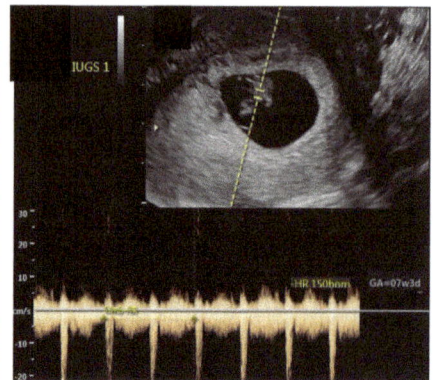

3.44f

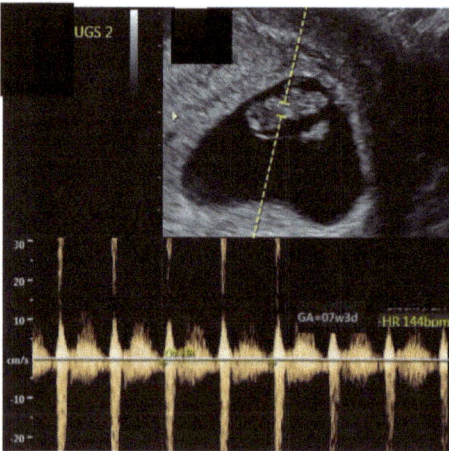

3.44f

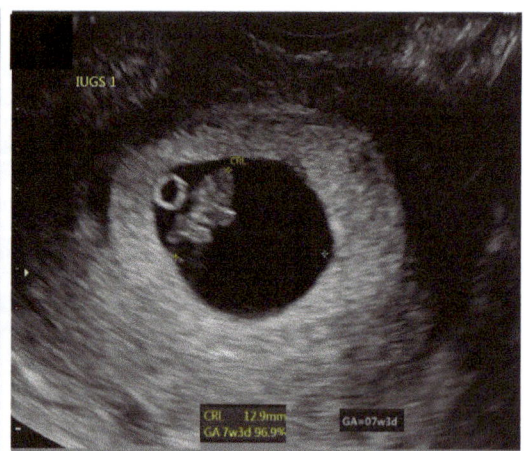

3.44g

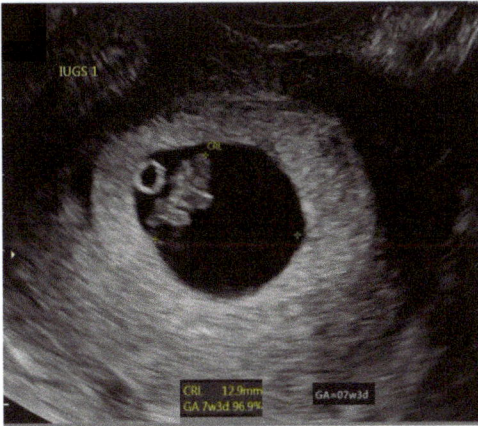

3.44h

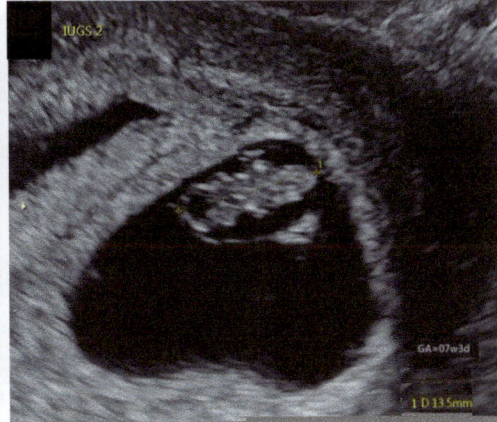

3.44i

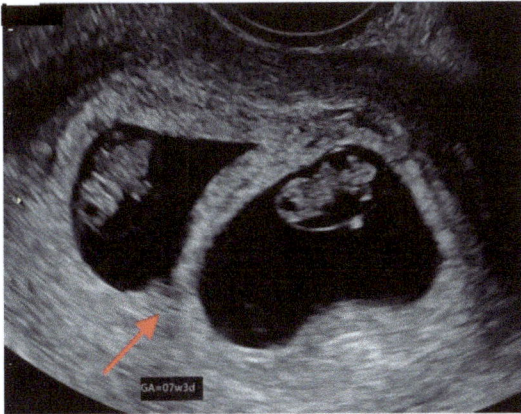

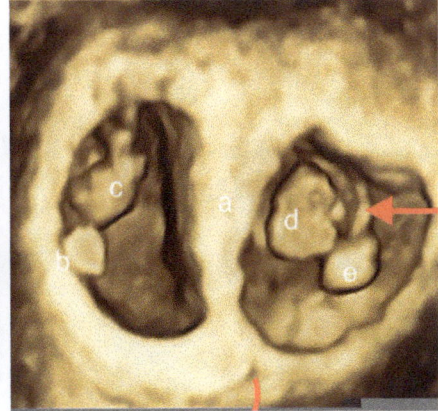

3.44j *Arrow –lambda sign*   **3.44k** *a-dividing membrane, b- yolk sac in the sac on the right, c- embryo in the sac on the right, d- embryo in the sac on the left, e- yolk sac in the sac on the left. Straight horizontal arrow – vitelline duct on the left, curved vertical arrow – lambda sign*
3.44l

IUGS 1	IUGS 2
GS – 23 x 20 x 24mm	GS – 25 x 28 x 26mm
YS - 4 x 4 x 6mm	YS - 5 x 5 x 6mm
CRL- 12.9mm	CRL- 13.5mm
FHB – 150bpm	FHB – 144bpm

Both ovaries not shown were enlarged with multiple corpus luteal cysts.
Impression: DCDA pregnancy

Pregnancy with generalised or local pelvic pain

Asking the patient to identify the area of pain prior and during the ultrasound examination is a useful tool that the sonographer should use. The sonographer can spend some time assessing the specified area to find the cause of pain.

3.45

This patient was referred with a history of bleeding and lower abdominal cramps at 10/40. She identified or located her pains to the bikini level. No EHB was seen.

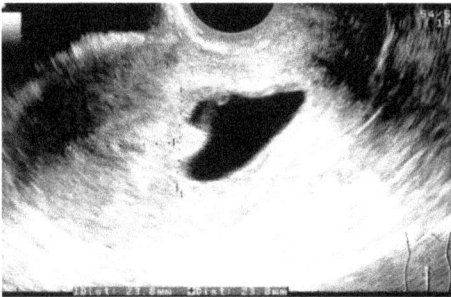

3.45a

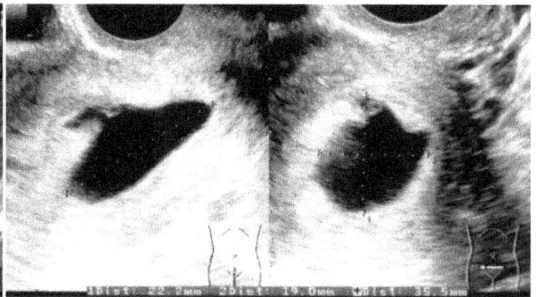

3.45b

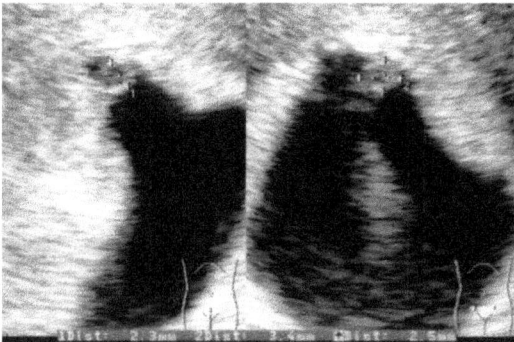

3.45c

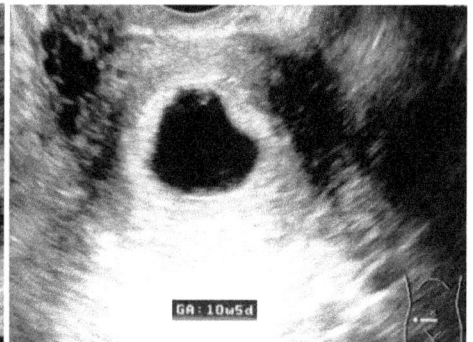

3.45d

Ultrasound finding: There is an irregular in outline gestational sac that is approx. 24mm from the uterine fundus (3.45a). Yolk sac seen, embryonic pole = 3.4mm and no EHB. There is an approx. 2 × 3 × 3mm echogenic triangular area in the fundal wall of this gestational sac (3.45a–b). ?polyp ?aetiology.

Impression: Ongoing missed abortion or miscarriage or ?cervical pregnancy.

Patients, in the process of miscarrying, often complain of intermittent crampy pains at the bikini level that precede some clotting or heavy bleeding after which they experience some relief.

  * Follow-up scan 7 days later revealed a complete miscarriage.

Chapter conclusion

The following are some of ultrasound indicators that are or may be predictive of poor prognosis or outcomes in the first trimester:

- Irregular in outline IUGS
- No FHB in CRL of > 5mm
- Abnormally large amniotic sac
- CRL that is less than expected
- Abnormal EHB/FHB **(see page 71)**
- Smaller IUGS than expected when compared to the embryo
- IUGS that implants not in the fundus but low in the cervix
- Eccentrically located gestational sac
- Abnormally large YS > 5.6mm in diameter in GA </=10/40
- Calcified or thick walled or irregular in outline YS
- Small GSV at less than 9/40 is associated with trisomy 16 and triploidy
- Poor IUGS growth. Normal growth rate is quoted as 1mm mean sac diameter per day
- Mean sac diameter minus CRL, that is, less than 5mm
- Gestational sac larger than 8mm without a YS or larger than 16mm without an embryo
- The presence of a subchorionic haematoma. It is believed that spontaneous loss rate in the presence of a subchorionic haematoma is increased in patients over the age of 35, and in a pregnancy that is less than 8 weeks' gestation
- Abnormal oedema around the fetal pole's abdomen or head
- Abnormal cystic entity in the fetal abdomen
- EHR rates below 100 bpm before 6.2 weeks and below 120 bpm at 6.3–7 weeks are associated with a significantly increased incidence of first-trimester pregnancy failure
- A slow EHB or FHR should be reported on the ultrasound report and a follow-up should be arranged to reassess the initial findings

Bibliography Chapters 3–4

Articles:

Abbasi S, Jamal A, Eslamian L, et al (2008) Role of Clinical and Ultrasound Findings in the Diagnosis of Retained Products of Conception. Available at: Ultrasound Obstetrics Gynecology 32(5): 704–707. doi: 10.1002/uog.5391

Abnormal Development – Ectopic Implantation. Available at: https://embryology.med.unsw.edu.au/embryology/index.

Ankum WM, Mol BW, der veen V, Bossuyt PM. (1996) Risk Factors for Ectopic Pregnancy: A Meta-analysis. Fertil Steril 65(6): 1093–1099. PubMed link

Bennett G L, Bromley B, Lieberman E, et al Subchorionic Hemorrhage in First-trimester Pregnancies: Prediction of Pregnancy Outcome with Sonography. Available at: http://pubs.rsna.org/doi/abs/10.1148/radiology.200.3.8756935

Bromley B, Shipp TD, Benacerraf BR. Structural Anomalies in Early Embryonic Death. http:www.jultrasoundmed.org/content/29/3/445. Full

Bromley B, Harlow BL, Laboda LA, et al (1991) Small Sac Size in the First trimester: A Predictor of Poor Fetal Outcome. Available at: Radiology 178: 375–377, 10.1148/radiology.178.2.1987595

Cerekja A. and Piazze J. Uterine Synechiae. Available at: http://sonoworld.com/fetus/page.aspx?id=2780

Chan LY1, Fok WY, Yuen PM. (2003) Pitfalls in Diagnosis of Interstitial Pregnancy. Available at: Acta Obstet Gynecol Scand 82(9): 867–870.

Chhabra A, Lin EC. Subchorionic Hemorrhage. Available at: http://emedicine.medscape.com/article/404971-overview

Confidential Enquiry into Maternal and Child Health (CEMACH) (2003–2005)

Reviewing Maternal Deaths to make Motherhood Safer. London.

Dhaliwal LK, Suri V, Gupta KR, et al (2011) Tamoxifen: An Alternative to Clomiphene in Women with Polycystic Ovary Syndrome. Available at: J Hum Reprod Sci 4(2): 76–79. Doi

Dighe M, Curvas C. (2008) Sonography in First-trimester Bleeding. J Clin Ultrasound 36(6): 352–366.

Durfee SM, Frates MC, Luong A, et al (2005) The Sonographic and Color Doppler Features of Retained Products of Conception. Available at: http://www.jultrasoundmed.org/content/24/9/1181.full 24(9): 1181–1186, quiz 1188–1189.

Early Pregnancy Information Centre. http://www.earlypregnancy.org.uk/index.asp

Ectopic Pregnancy and Miscarriage: Diagnosis and Initial Management in Early Pregnancy of Ectopic Pregnancy and Miscarriage. http://www.nice.org.uk/guidance/CG154

Fadhlaoui A, Khrouf M, Khémiri K, et al. (2012) Successful Conservative Treatment of a Cesarean Scar Pregnancy with Systemically Administered Methotrexate and Subsequent Dilatation and Curettage: A Case Report. Available at: Case Reports in Obstetrics and Gynecology, Article ID 248564, 6 pagesdoi:10.1155/2012/248564

Farooq S et al. Uterine leiomyoma Available at: https://radiopaedia.org/articles/uterine-leiomyoma

Farquharson R. Guidelines 2007 of Association of Early Pregnancy Units. Available at http://www.ptmp.com.pl/archives/apm/13-4/APM134-guidelines-7-28.pdf

Fong KW, Toi A, Salem S, Hornberger, et al Detection of Fetal Structural

Abnormalities with US during Early Pregnancy. Available at: http://radiographics.rsna.org/conten6/24/1/157.full?sid

Gibson CM, Dmello M. Hydatidiform Mole. Available at: http://wikidoc.org/index.php/Hydatidiform_mole

http://www. bcshguidelines.com/documents/Neonatal/GuidelineFinalNov2010.pdf

http://www.nhs.uk/Conditions/Haemophilia/Pages/Introduction.aspx

Hyperemesis Gravidarum. Available at: http://www.whattoexpect.com/pregnancy/pregnancy-health/complications/hyperemesis-gravidarum.aspx

Hyperemesis Gravidarum. Available at: http://americanpregnancy.org/pregnancy-complications/hyperemesis-gravidarum

Karaer A, Avsar FA, Batioglu S. (2006) Risk Factors for Ectopic Pregnancy: A Case-control Study. Aust N Z J Obstet Gynaecol 46(6): 521–527. PubMed link.

Lau WL, Cahn LL, Chan KS, et al 3D-Ultrasound Diagnosis of the Cervical Pregnancy. Available at: http://www.sonoworld.com/fetus/page.aspx?id=3013

Lefebvre G, Vilos G, Allaire C, Jeffrey J, et al (2003) The management of uterine leiomyomas. J Obstet Gynaecil Can 25(5): 396–418, quiz 419–422.

Morin L, Van den Hof MC. Ultrasound Evaluation of First-trimester Pregnancy Complications. Available at: http://sogc.org/wp-content/uploads/2013/01/161E-CPG-June2005.pdf

Moustafa MR and Burnham A. (2009) Conservative Management of Multiple Ovarian Pregnancy. BMUS Ultrasound 17(1): 35–36.

Nicol M. (2009 June) Reporting On: Gynecological Ultrasound. Synergy Imaging &

Therapy Practice

Ogunyemi DA and Isaacs C. Hyperemesis Gravidarum. Available at: http://emedicine.medscape.com/article/254751-overview

Peel A. (2009) Diagnosis of An Intestitial Ectopic Pregnancy with Two-Dimensional Transvaginal Sonography. BMUS Ultrasound 17(2): 93–95.

Raheem M, Abukhalil I. (2005) Ectopic Pregnancy - An Update. The Middle East Journal of Emergency Medicine. 5(1).

Ramsey E & Shilitto J. (2008) How Early Can Fetal Heart Pulsations Be Detected Reliably Using Modern Ultrasound Equipment? BMUS Ultrasound 16(4): 193–195.

Reichman D, Laufer MR, Robinson BK, et al. Pregnancy Outcomes in Unicornuate Uteri: A review. Fertility and Sterility 91(5): 1886–1894. doi:10.1016/j.fertnstert.2008.02.163. PMID 18439594

Royal College of Obstetricians and Gynaecologists (2006) The Management of Early Pregnancy Loss. Green-top Guideline, no. 25. London.

Royal College of Obstetricians and Gynaecologists (2011 April) The Investigation and Treatment of Couples with Recurrent First-trimester and Second-trimester Miscarriage. Green–top Guideline, no. 17. London RCOG. Available at: https://www.rcog.org.uk/globalassets/documents/guidelines/gtg_17.pdf

Sagili H and Mohamed K. (2008) Pregnancy of Unknown Location: An evidence-based approach to management. The Obstetrician & Gynecologist 10: 224–230.

Shah C, Johnson PT, Bhanushali A, et al. Complete Molar Gestation: Role of Ultrasound. Available at: http://www.sonoworld.com/ArticleDetails/CompleteMolar_Gestation_Role_of_Ultrasound.aspx?ArticleId=15

Shah C, Johnson PT, Gianc P. Partial Molar Gestation: Available at: http://www.sonoworld.com/ArticleDetails/Partial_Molar_Gestation_Rol

Sheth S. Cornual (Interstitial) Ectopic Pregnancy. Available at: http://sonoworld.com/CaseDetails/Cornual_(interstitial)_ectopic_pregnancy.aspx?ModuleCategoryId=263

Skandhan AKP and Radswiki, et al. Atypical Ectopic Pregnancy. Available at: http://radiopaedia.org/articles/atypical-ectopic-pregnancy

Venkatakrishnan H. Ultrasound During Pregnancy. Available at: http://www.medindia.net/patients/patientinfo/ultrasound-during-pregnancy.htm

Vohra S, Mahsood S, Shelton H, et al.
Spontaneous Live Unilateral Twin Ectopic Pregnancy – A Case Presentation
Available at: http://ult.sagepub.com/content/22/4/243

Weiss RE. (2014) Molar Pregnancy. Available at: http://pregnancy.about.com/od/cancerinpregnanc/a/Molar-Pregnancy.htm

Worrall JA and Dubose T. (2011) Recognizing Intra-amniotic Band-like Structures on Obstetric Ultrasound. Available at:
www.obgyn.net/articles/recognizing-intra-amniotic-band-structures-obstetric-ultrasound.

Chapter 4

Case presentations

Some case presentations of the use of ultrasound in early pregnancy will be presented in this chapter.

4.1

This patient was referred because of light vaginal bleeding for 3/7 prior to this scan. The right ovary was not visualised but the left ovary (not shown here) appeared sonographically normal. No ultrasound abnormality was seen in the pelvis.

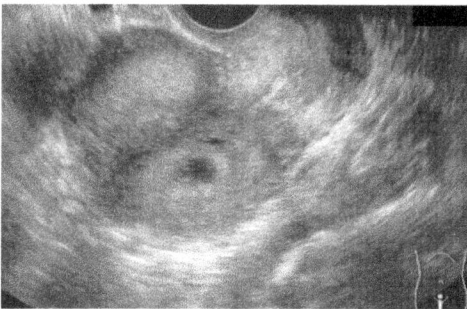

4.1a

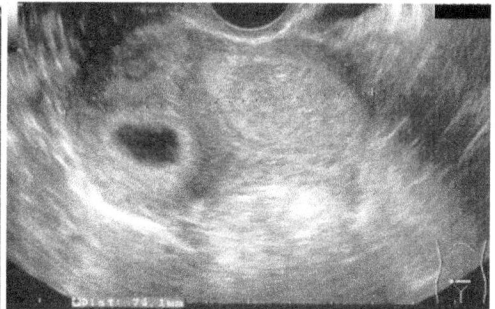

4.1b

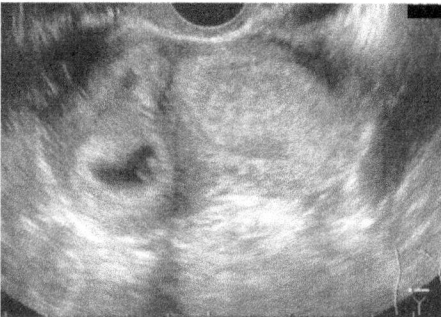

4.1c

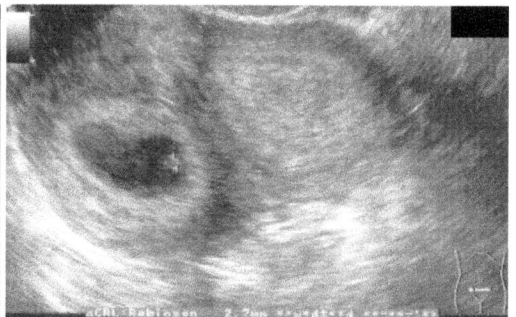

4.1d

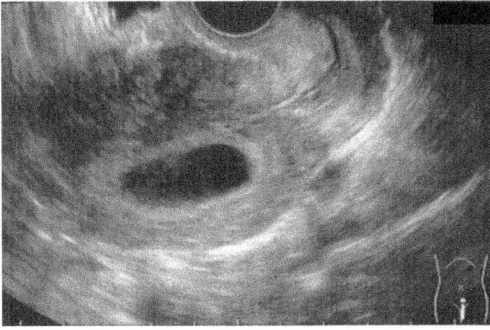

4.1e

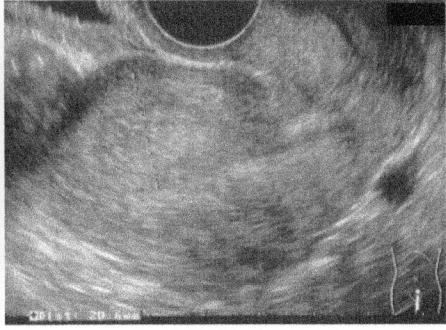

4.1f

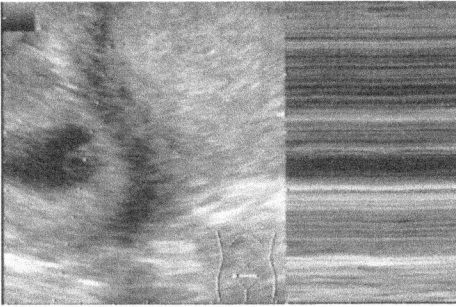

4.1g

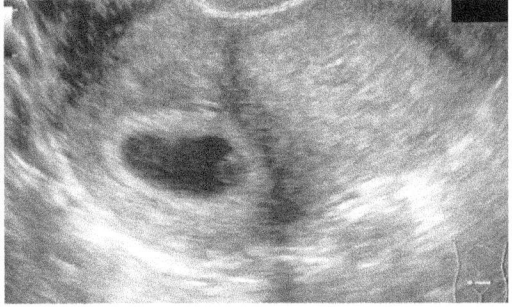

4.1h

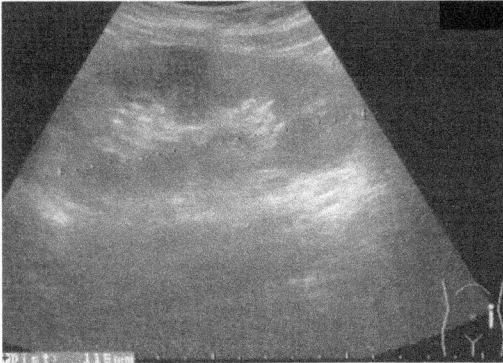

4.1i

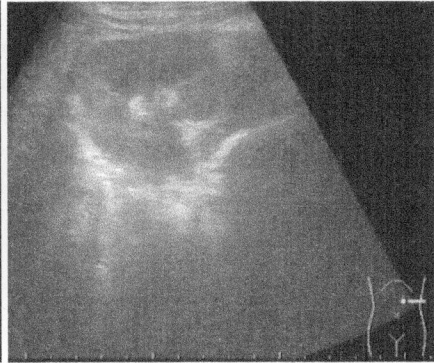

4.j

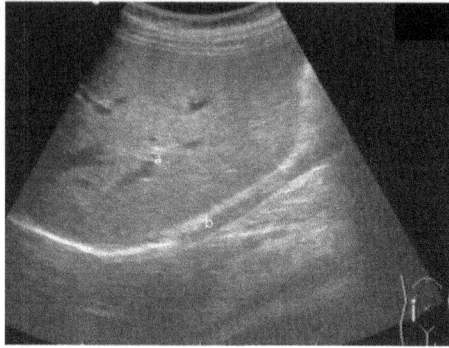

4.1k *a-liver, b- missing right kidney in the renal bed*

Ultrasound findings: Bicornuate uterus with one cervix (4.1a–f), the pregnancy is in the right horn (4.1c, e, h). Singleton intrauterine pregnancy. YS, fetal pole, EHB seen (4.1a–h), CRL = 2.7mm (4.1d). The left endometrial thickness is 27mm (4.1f). The pv. bleeding is most likely from the decidual reaction in the left horn.

There is no kidney in the expected right renal bed or in the pelvis (4.1k arrow showing liver). There is a normal looking left kidney measuring approx.11.5cm in length (4.1i-j).

The patient was not aware that she had only one kidney

The pregnancy progressed normally

Patients with uterine abnormalities have been reported to have urinary tract anomalies in about 40% of cases, including ectopic kidney, renal agenesis, double renal pelvis, horseshoe kidneys and unilateral medullary sponge kidney

4.2

This patient was sent to empty her urinary bladder pre TVS. She returned more than 10 minutes later and here are the ultrasound findings. CRL = expected GA.

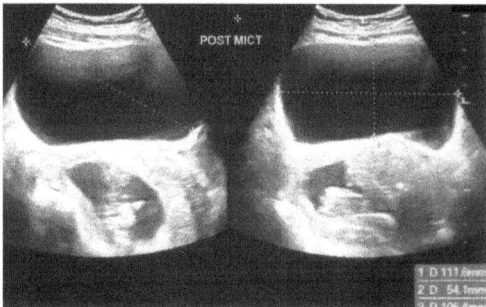
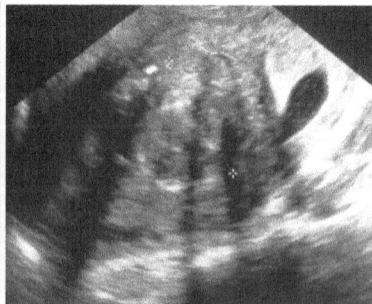

4.2a   **4.2b** (32 × 37 × 32mm)

Ultrasound findings: Retroverted uterus with an IUP. Significant post void volume. (11.6 × 5.4 × 10.6 × 0.7 = 464.8ml – (4.2a). Retroverted uterus with an IUP. There is an anterior cervical fibroid measuring approx. 32 × 37 × 32mm (4.2b).

There was another fibroid (not shown here)

See chapter 3 for more on fibroids in pregnancy

4.3

This is a follow-up scan in a patient who had a history of pv. bleeding in this pregnancy.

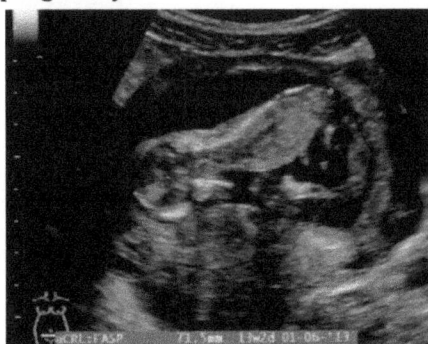
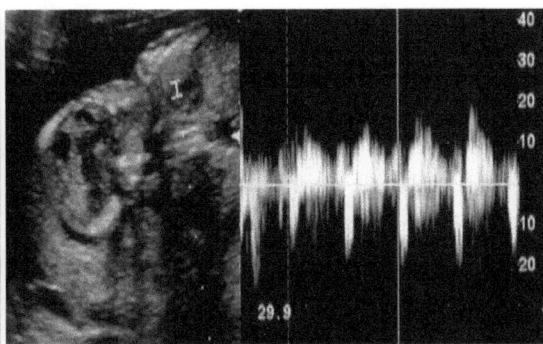

4.3a   **4.3b** FHR – 155bpm

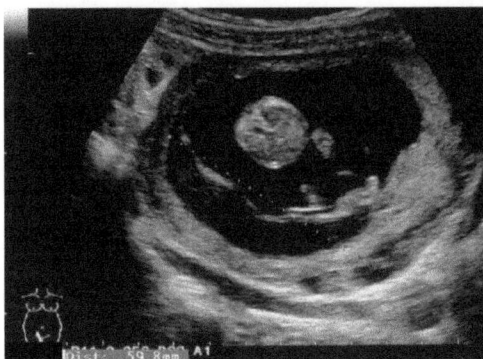
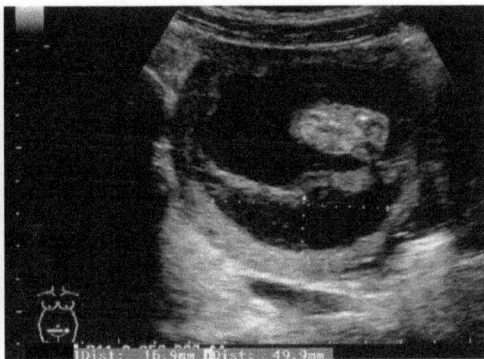

4.3c   **4.3d**

Ultrasound findings: Single intrauterine gestational sac, fetus with FHB of 155bpm (4.3b). CRL = 72mm = 13+2 (4.3a). There is posterior subchorionic haematoma measuring approx. 60 × 50 × 17mm (4.3c–d).

Impression: Subchorionic haematoma. The differential diagnosis is uterine synechiae, but this condition does not present with pv. bleeding. The endometrium was regular and the same thickness throughout. It was too thick, irregular and of various thicknesses to be an unfused amnion.

* It is believed that late first- or second-trimester subchorionic haematoma carries a worse prognosis than if the haematoma develops earlier in the pregnancy.

4.4

This patient was referred for a scan because she was experiencing the 'bikini line' pains.

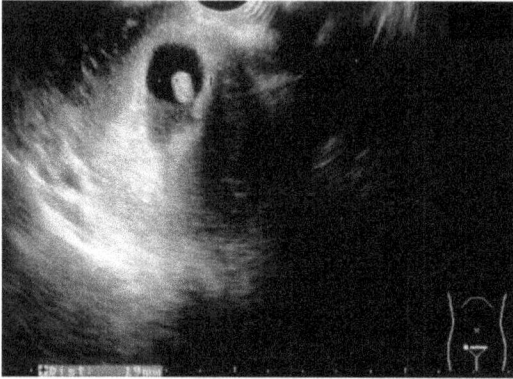

4.4a

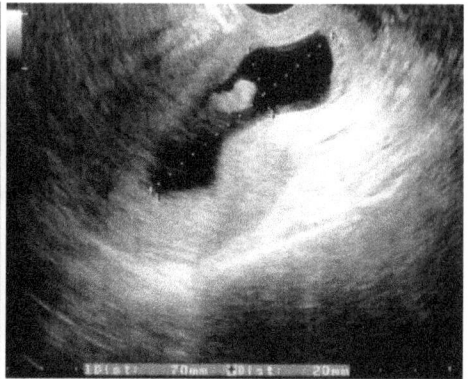

4.4b

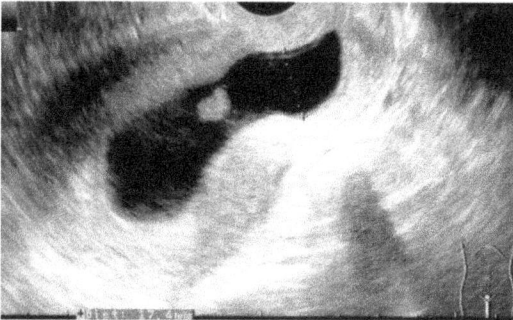

4.4c

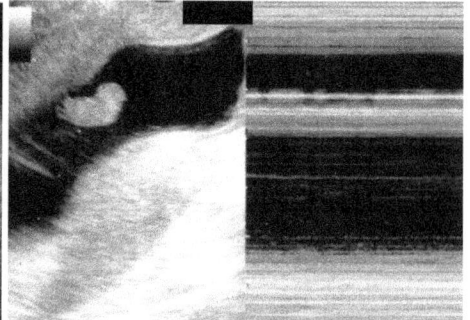

4.4d

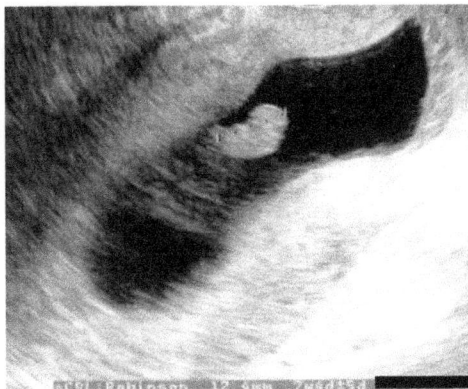

4.4e

Ultrasound findings: Elongated, irregular in outline gestational sac (4.4b–e). There is an embryo with no EHB and almost at the internal os (4.4b–e). CRL = 12.4mm = 7+4/40 (4.4e). Internal os is opened (4.4b, d–e)

Impression: Inevitable abortion/ongoing miscarriage.

* The patient subsequently miscarried.

4.5

This patient was referred for a follow-up scan at 5/40 GA.

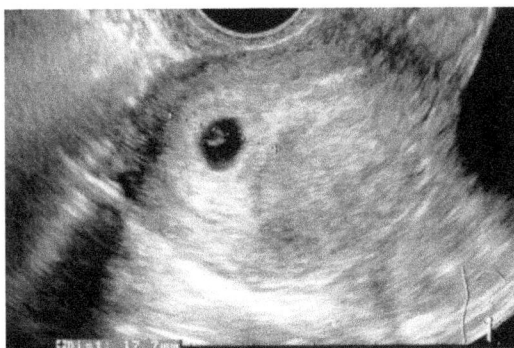 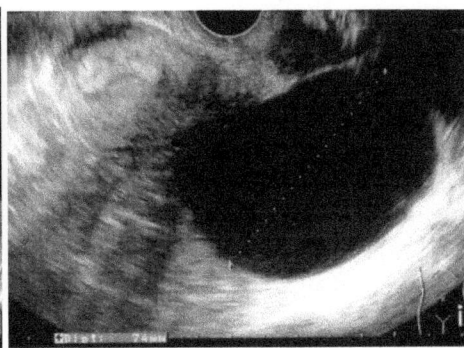

4.5a   **4.5b**

GSV = 0.4ml.

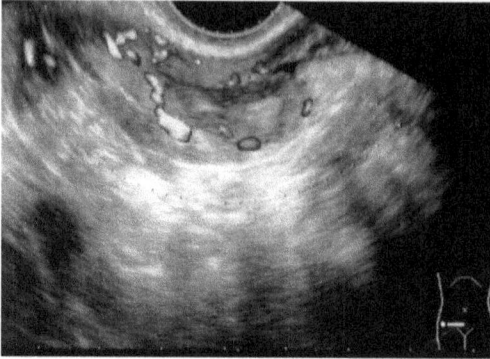

4.5c

Note the 'ring of fire'.

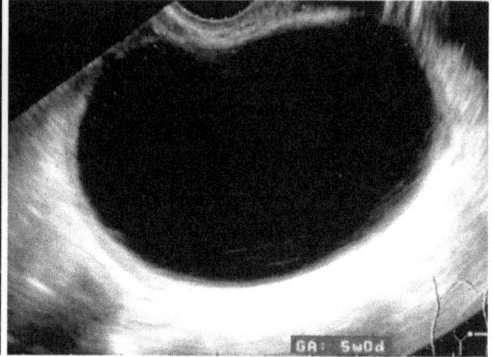

4.5d

No vascularity around this cyst

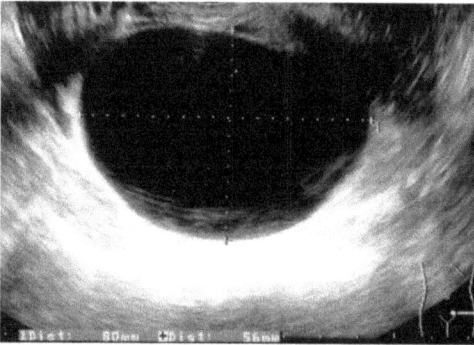

4.5e

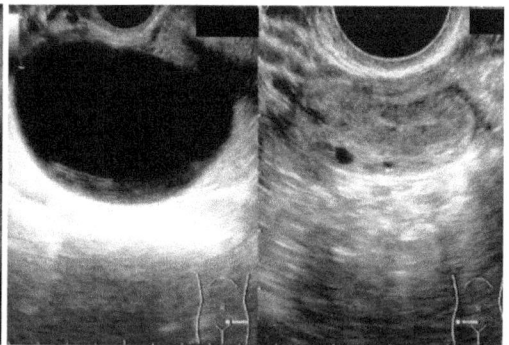

4.5f

Ultrasound findings: An IUGS and YS. No embryonic pole is demonstrated (4.5a). There is a CLC on the right (4.5c). There is an approx. 74 × 80 × 56mm avascular cystic entity posterior to the uterus and on the left (4.5b, d–f). There is some ovarian tissue in the lateral wall of this cyst. The left ovary (not shown) is separate from this cystic entity.

Impression: An early IUP appropriate for GA. CLC on the right and an avascular cyst on the left. A follow-up scan (in 2–3 weeks), with the intention of dating the pregnancy and re-assessing the cystic entity on the left, is recommended.

It is important that the left cystic entity be checked at a subsequent ultrasound examination and measured to establish if it grows or otherwise

*Should this patient develop LIF pains in the pregnancy, an ovarian torsion will have to be excluded as the cause of the pain.

4.6

This patient was scanned as a follow-up at 8+6/40. Previous scan was at 6+4/40 where it was noted that the GSD was below the fifth centile for that GA.

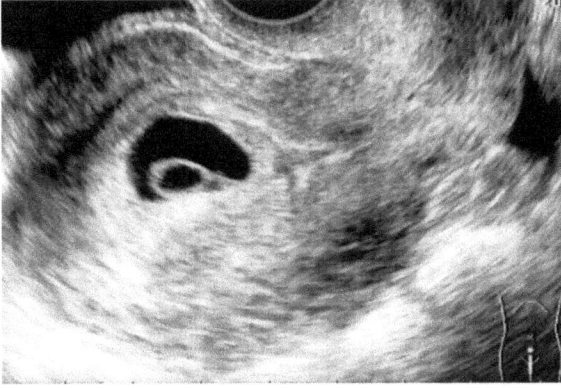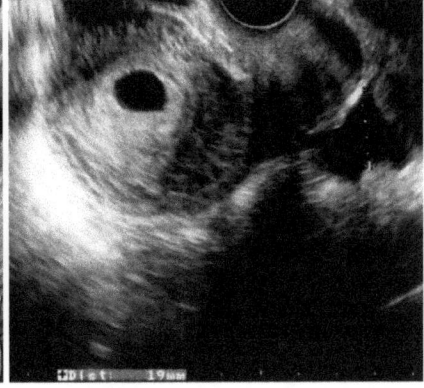

| 4.6a. | 4.6b. |

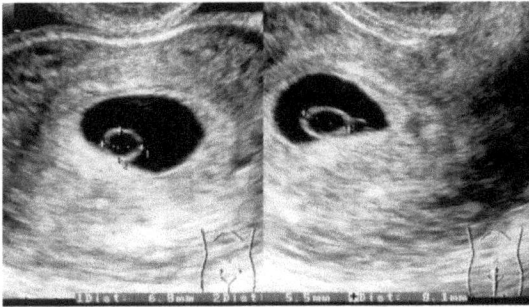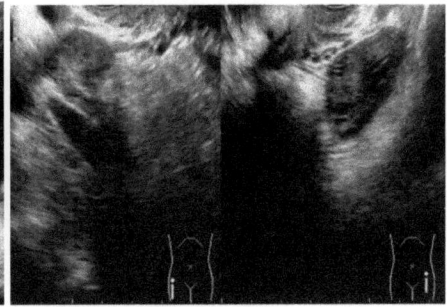

| 4.6c | 4.6d |

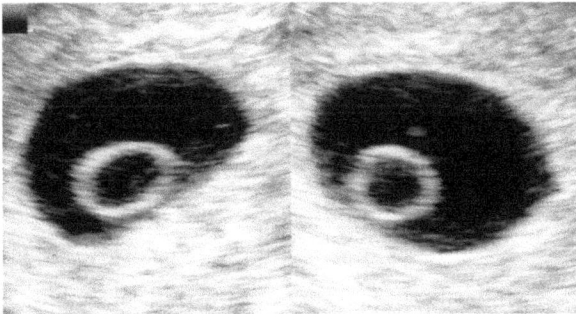

4.6e

Ultrasound findings: IUGS (4.6a–b) with a yolk sac measuring 7 × 6 × 8mm

(4.6c) but no obvious fetal pole. YS above the 95th centile for GA. GSD still less than the fifth centile for GA. Tiny possible area of bleeding to the right of the GS. Some anechoic fluid in the POD up to 19mm (4.6a–b). Both ovaries have normal morphology with no obvious CLC (4.6d). The ovarian measurements have not been included.

Impression: Inconclusive. Suggest a follow-up scan 7–10 days from then.

*At the next follow-up scan patient miscarried.

4.7

This patient was referred at 11/40 with a 3/7 history of bleeding. Both ovaries (not shown) appeared sonographically normal. AP endometrial measurement was 27mm. Below is the TS view of the uterus.

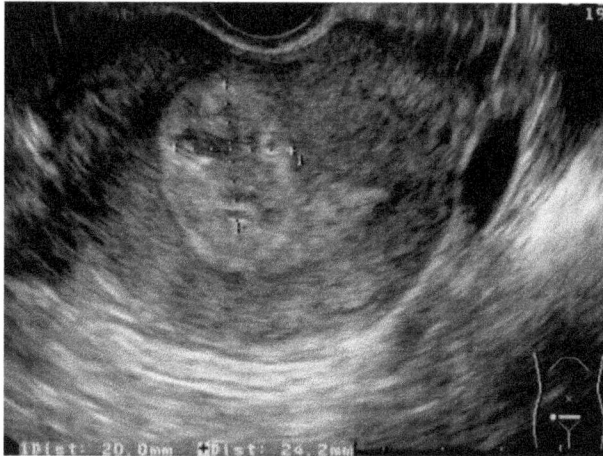

4.7a

Ultrasound findings: No obvious IUGS seen. RPOC seen in the endometrium measuring approx. 27 × 20 × 24mm. The endometrium is 27mm thick.

Impression: RPOC in the endometrium.

4.8

This patient was scanned at 8+6/40 as a follow-up scan for dating. Previous scan was at 6/40. Left ovary (not shown here) appeared sonographically normal. The right ovary was not identified.

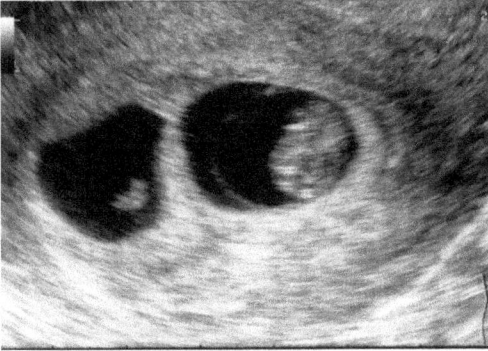

4.8a

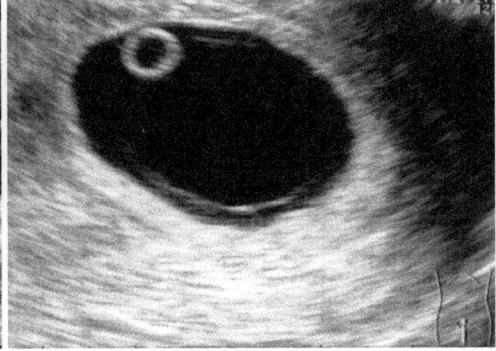

4.8b

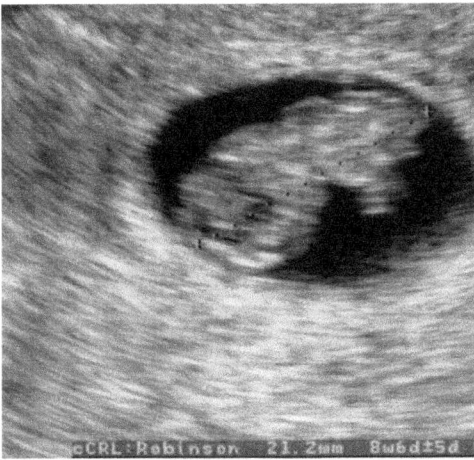

4.8c

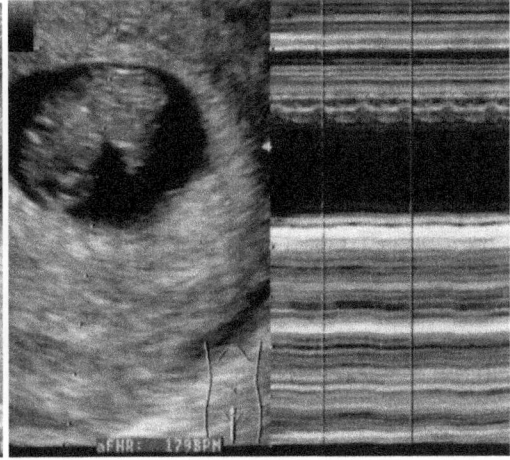

4.8d

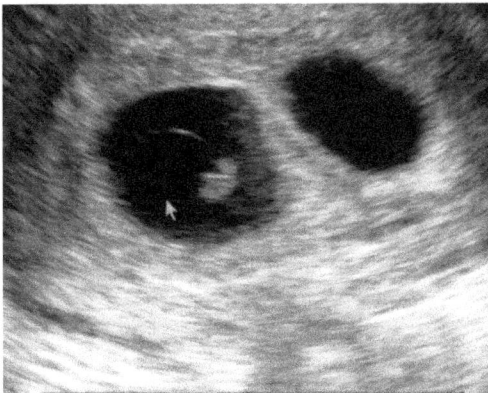

4.8e

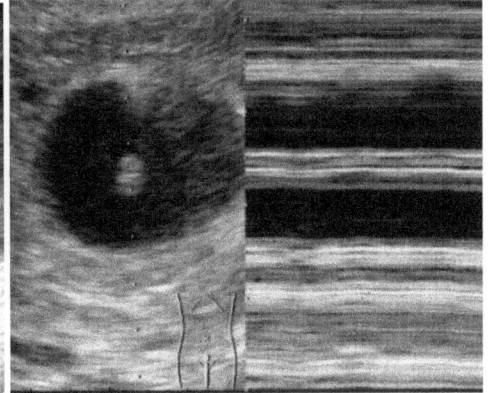

4.8f

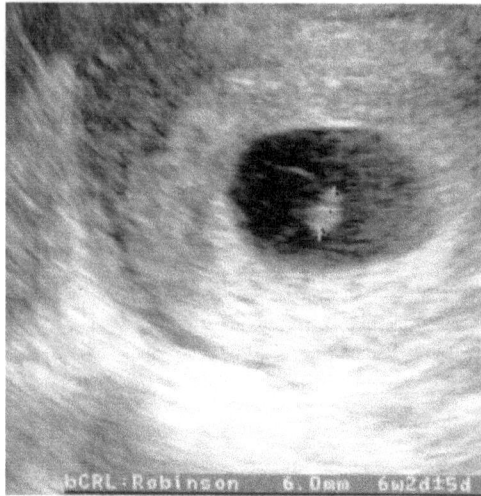

4.8g

Ultrasound findings: Two IUGs (4.8a & e). GS 1 is on maternal left. GS, EP with EHB is seen. EHR = 177bpm. CRL = 21mm = 8+6/40 (4.8c–d).

GS 2 is on maternal right. GS is slightly irregular in outline, YS and FP present. No FHB. CRL = 6mm (4.8a, e–g).

Impression: DC/DA Twins. No FHB in GS 2. = Missed abortion or miscarriage. EP in GS 1 – Ongoing pregnancy.

*At follow-up scan appointments, this will be treated as a single pregnancy.

4.9

This patient was referred with a history of pv. bleeding at 5+5/40. Both ovaries (not shown) appeared sonographically normal.

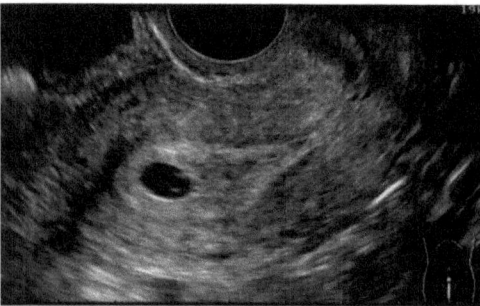
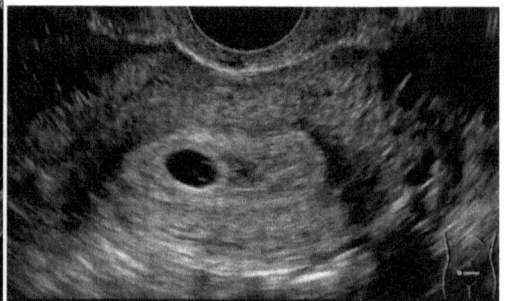

| **4.9a** | **4.9b** |

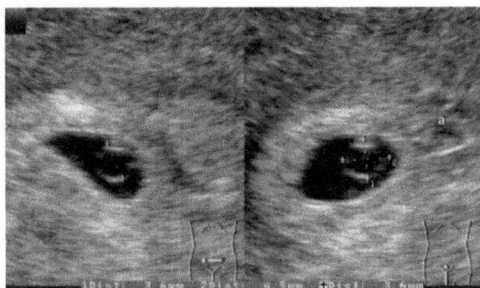 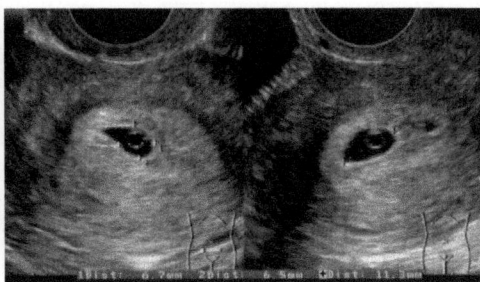

4.9c   **4.9d**

a- ? a small predominantly hypoechoic area adjacent to b

Ultrasound findings: An IUGS and a YS (4.9a–d). No embryonic pole is identified. IUGS measuring 11 × 7 × 7mm. GSD = 1.1 × 0.7 × 0.7 × 0.5233 = 0.3ml (4.9.d). YS measuring 4 × 4.4 × 5mm (4.9.c). To the left of the GS is a small predominantly hypoechoic area (4.9c) (measurements are not included).

Impression: An early IUP with a small area of bleeding possibly an implantational bleed. Suggest a dating scan in 2–3 weeks.

* Follow-up – Normal ongoing pregnancy.

4.10

This patient was referred at 6+4/40 with a history of spotting in early pregnancy.

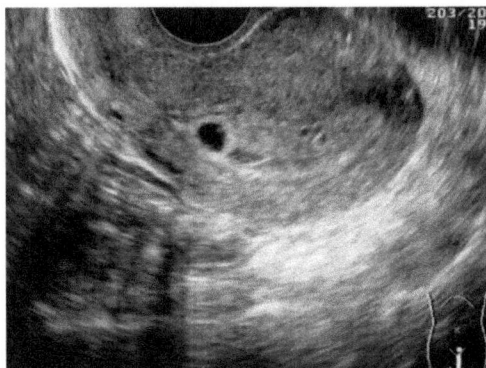 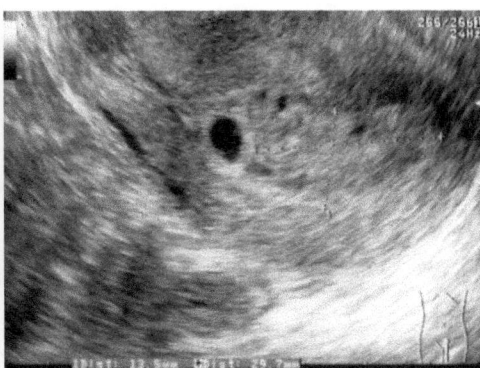

4.10a   **4.10b**

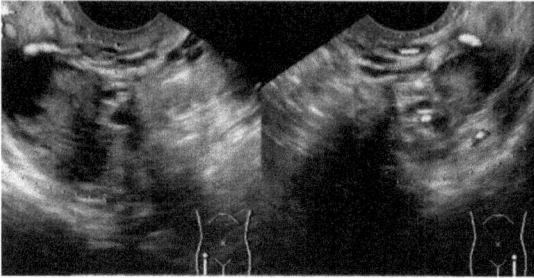

4.10c

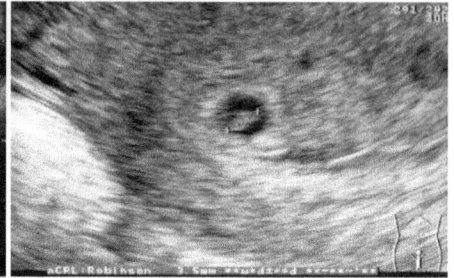

4.10d

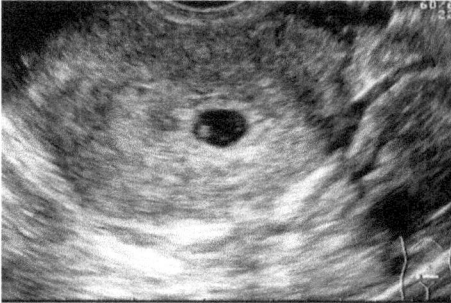

4.10e

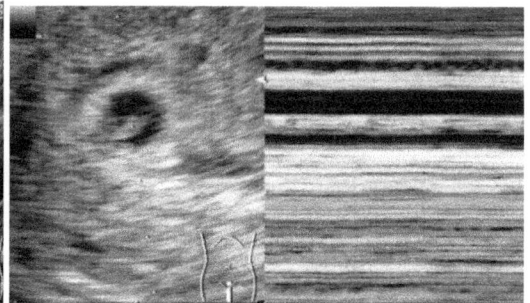

4.10f

Ultrasound findings: R/V uterus (4.10a–b). An IUGS with a YS, EP and EHB is seen. CRL = 3.5mm (d, e–f). There is a possible small area of bleeding around the sac (4.10f). The IUGS is approx. 30mm from the fundus.

Impression: IUGS that is approx. 30mm from the fundus. ? eccentric location.

4.11

This patient was referred as a follow-up. Right ovary (not shown) appeared normal. The left ovary was not identified.

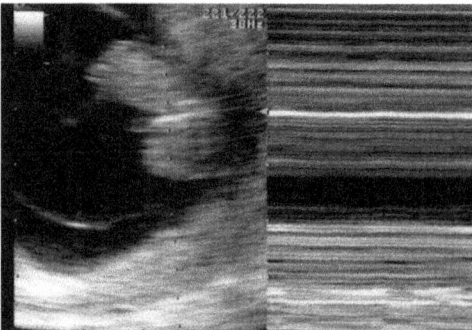

4.11a

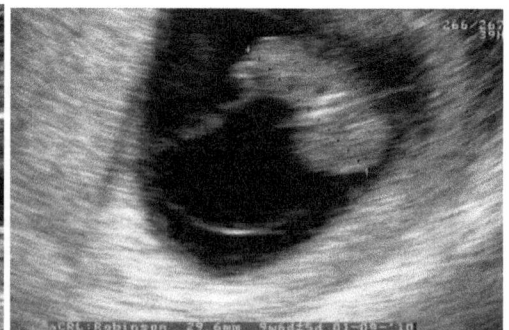

4.11b

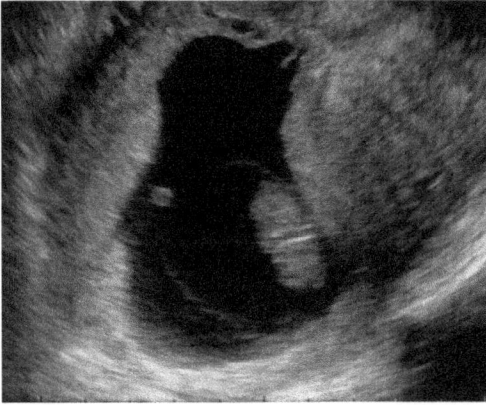 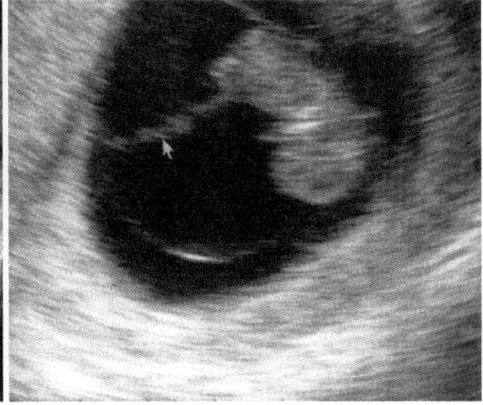

4.11c   **4.11d**

Arrow showing the umbilical cord.

Ultrasound findings: An irregular in outline IUGS with a YS,
fetal pole (4.11c, a–b) that does not have any FHB (4.11a). CRL = 30mm = 9+6/40
(4.11b).

Impression: Missed abortion or miscarriage.

4.12

This patient was known to have a partial septated uterus. She was referred
at 6+6/40 with a history of light vaginal bleeding for 17 days. She had three
previous miscarriages @ < 15/40.

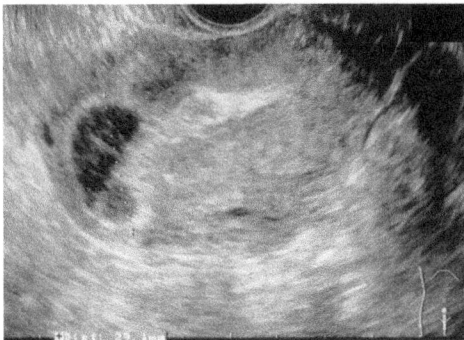 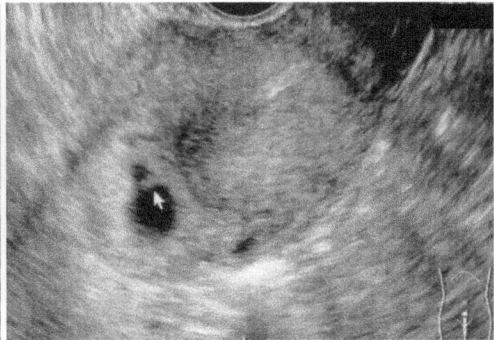

4.12a   **4.12b**

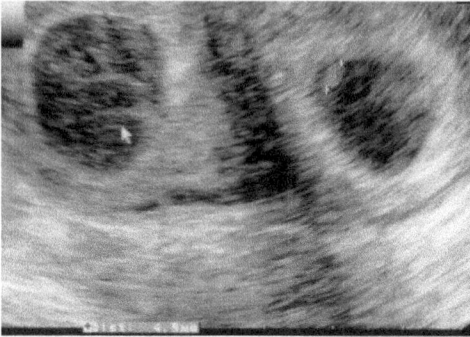
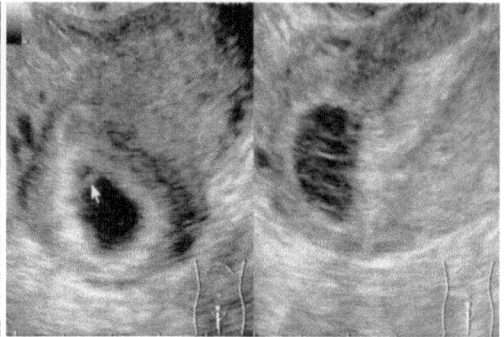

4.12c   **4.12d**

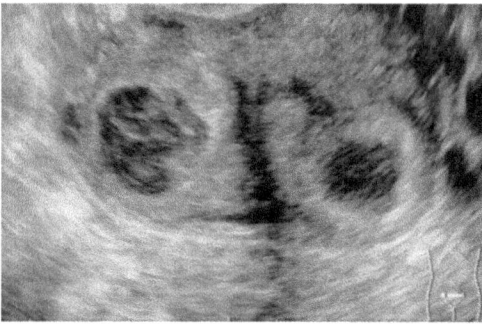
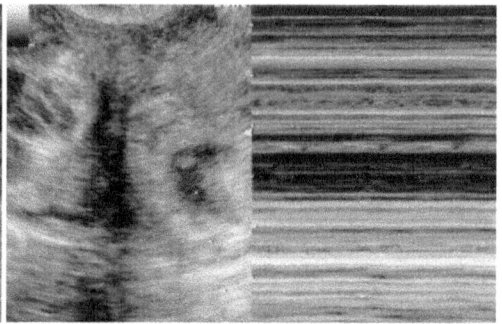

4.12e   **4.12f**

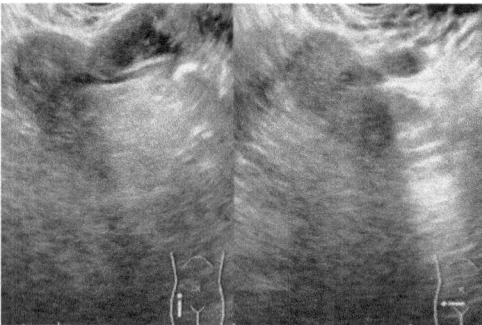
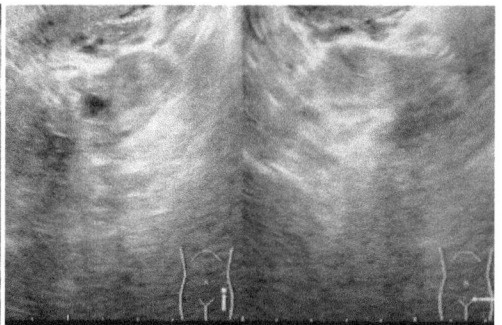

4.12g   **4.12h**

Ultrasound findings: Septated uterus with an EP in the left horn (4.12d) CRL = 4.5mm (4.12c). The right horn is filled with a haemorrhagic collection which perhaps explains the patient's ongoing and prolonged pv. bleeding (4.12a). The right ovary appears sonographically normal (4.12g), whilst there is a small corpus luteum in the left ovary (4.12h).

Impression: Septated uterus with an EP and EHB. However, because the CRL is <

GA by LMP, a follow-up or dating scan is recommended.

* It is believed that 8–23% of women who experience a recurrent miscarriage will have some form of uterine malformation, a third of these women with uterine malformation will have a septate uterus.

* In a patient with a septate uterus, there is a band of tissue or septum that is in the middle of her uterus. It is believed that there is poor blood supply to this septum and that pregnancies that implant on the septum are at a higher risk of miscarriage as the placenta cannot develop properly and access nutrients. Those who do not miscarry may be at increased risk of preterm labour and of having a premature baby.

* A septate uterus is a congenital abnormality or malformation; it should be distinguished from a bicornuate uterus.

* The miscarriage rate in women with septate uteri is quoted as between 25 and 47%.

4.13
This patient was referred with a history of LIF pains with a positive pregnancy test at 5+5/40.

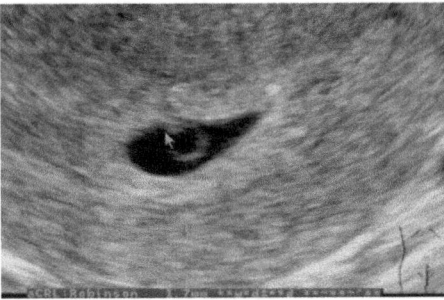 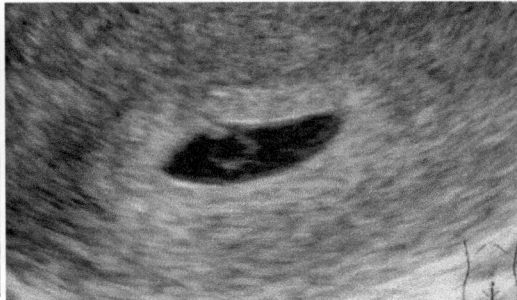

4.13a	**4.13b**

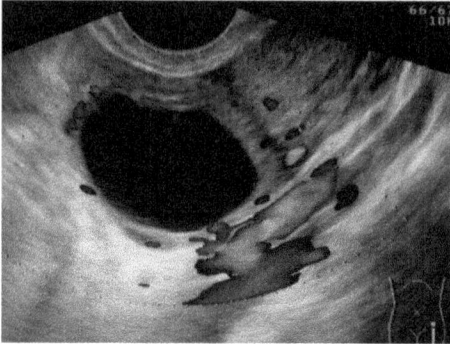
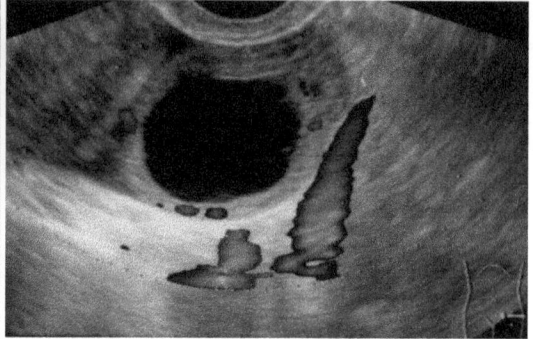

4.13c   **4.13d**

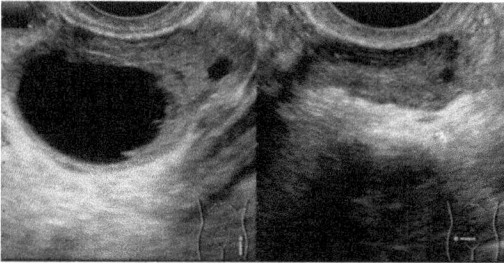
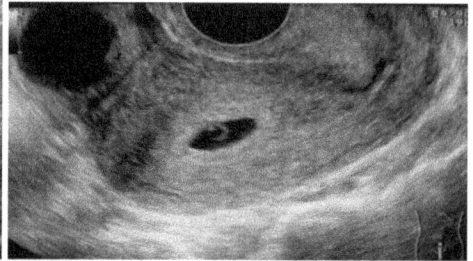

4.13e   **4.13f**

Ultrasound findings: Single intrauterine gestational sac, YS, no fetal pole seen yet (4.13a–b, f). There is a corpus luteum in the left ovary (4.13c–e). (measurements not included). The right ovary appears sonographically normal (4.13e image on the right)

*The cyst was seen in the area of the patient's pain.

Impression: Corpus luteum in the area of the patient's pain. Suggest a dating scan 2–3 weeks later.

4.14

This patient was referred with a history of brownish discharge in pregnancy.

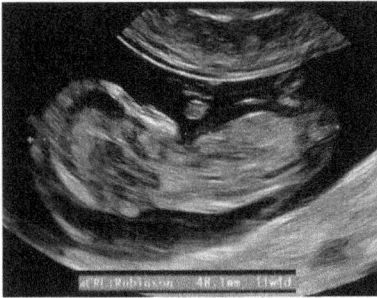
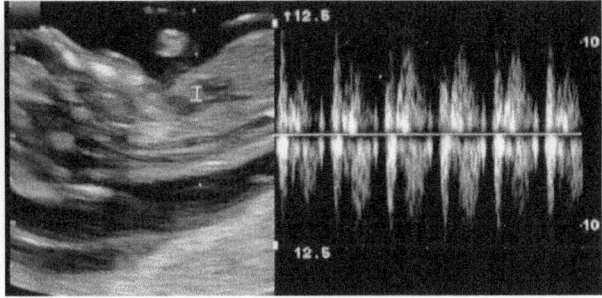

4.14a　　　　　　　　　　**4.14b**

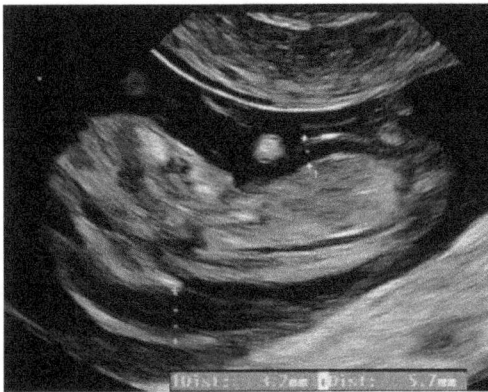
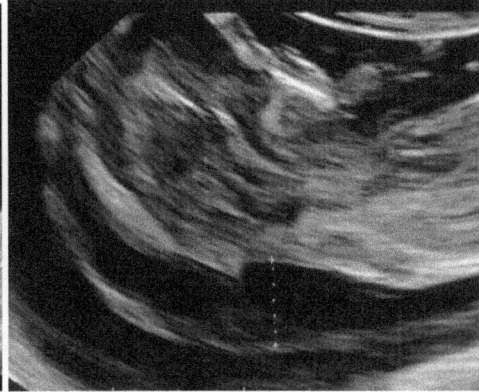

4.14c　　　　　　　　　　**4.14d**

Ultrasound findings: Single intrauterine gestational sac and fetus with FHB (4.14.a-b). CRL = 48.1mm = 11+4/40 (4.14a). There is fetal hydrops (4.14c) and increased NT (4.14c &.d).

Impression: Fetal hydrops and will need further fetal assessment.

Some days later:

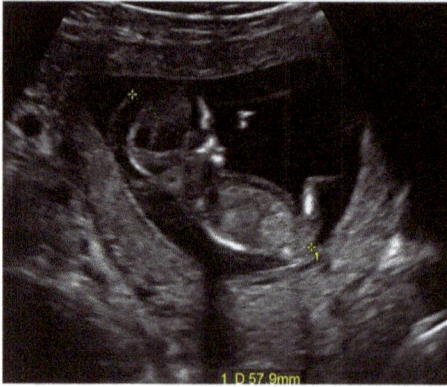

4.14e

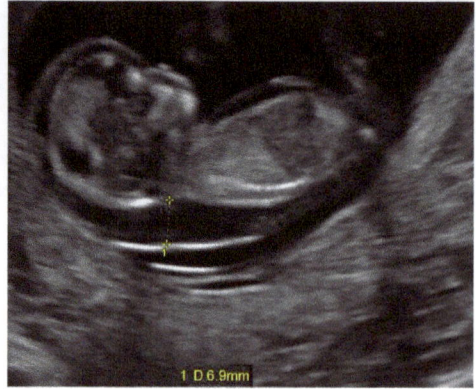

4.14f

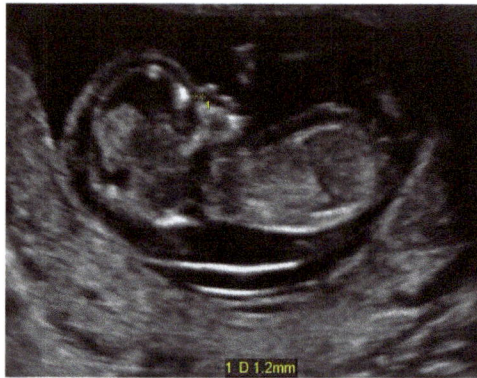

4.14g

* Follow-up scans as above confirmed fetal hydrops and increased NT (4.14e–g). Single umbilical artery was also noticed.

4.15

This patient was referred with a history of abdominal pain. She delivered a baby 4 months earlier and had only two periods before this pregnancy. Considerable overlying bowel gas was seen in the area of the patient's pain. By her LMP, GA should be 7+4/40, but the patient thought she was 4/40 pregnant.

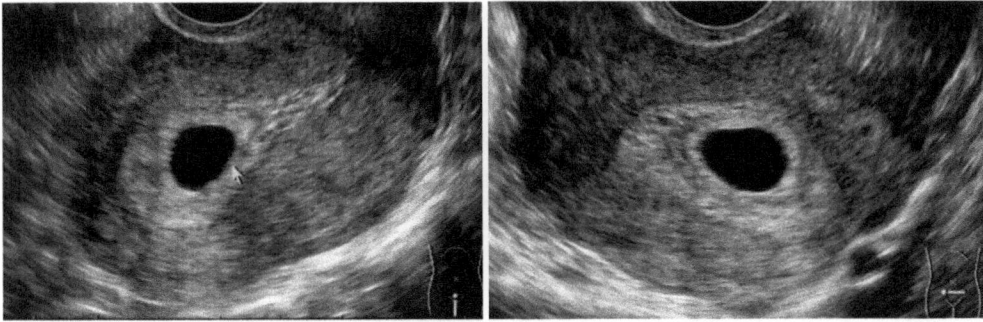

4.15a   4.15b

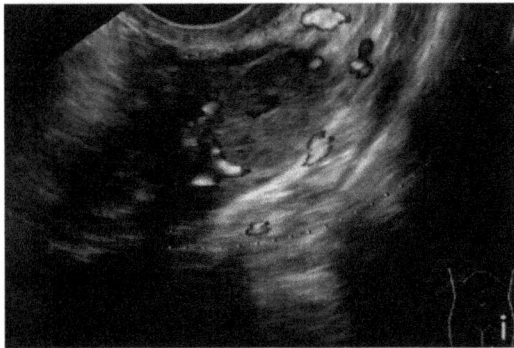

4.15c

Ultrasound findings: An IUGS but no YS or EMP yet (4.15a–b). IUGS measurement has not been included. There is a corpus luteum cyst in the left ovary (4.15c). Right ovary not included.

Impression: An early IUGS. Suggest a follow-up scan in 7–10 days from this scan. GIT problems cannot be excluded in view of the bowel gas in the area of patient's pain. A co-existing ectopic pregnancy is unlikely in this patient because it is a natural conception and one corpus luteum has been demonstrated.

*Follow-up: Ongoing singleton pregnancy but less than LMP date.

4.16

This patient was referred with a history of ?SROM at 16+2/40. HC = GA.

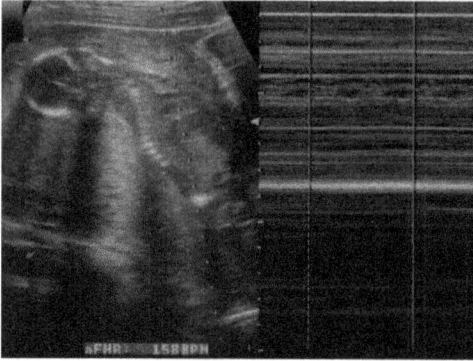

4.16a

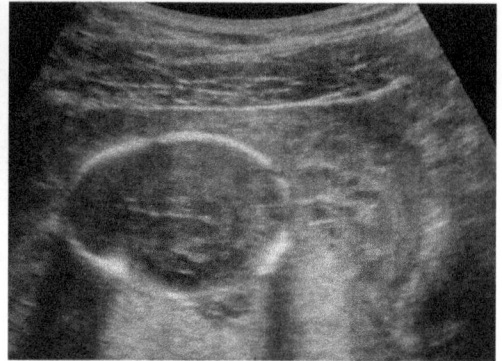

4.16b

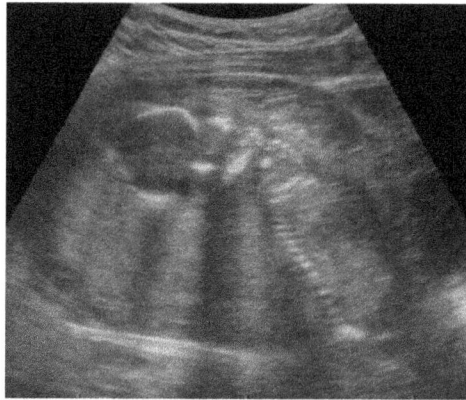

4.16c

Ultrasound findings: Single intrauterine pregnancy (4.16a–b). FHB seen (4.16a). Breech presentation. Anhydramnios. Posterior placenta not low (4.16c). Fetal anatomy cannot be assessed in view of anhydramnios.

Impression: Anyhdramnios. Single intrauterine pregnancy.

*Though this fetus was alive at the time of the scan, the prognosis is bad.

* This is an example of conveying bad news to the patient or couple.

* Patient later miscarried.

Some causes of oligo or anhydramnios include the following:

- SROM
- PROM
- Placental insufficiency
- High blood pressure

- Congenital malformation or blockage of baby's urinary tract, e.g. renal agenesis, polycystic kidneys and obstruction of the urinary tract
- Congenital heart defect

4.17

This patient was referred for a follow-up scan at 7+2/40 with a history of one gestational sac smaller than the other. EHB x 2 (not shown here) were seen.

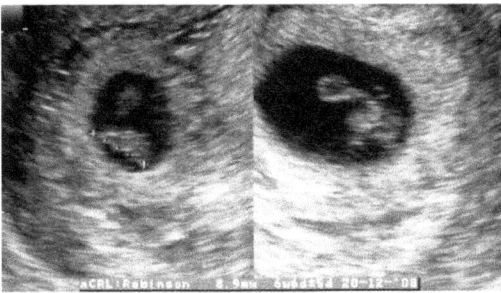

4.17a

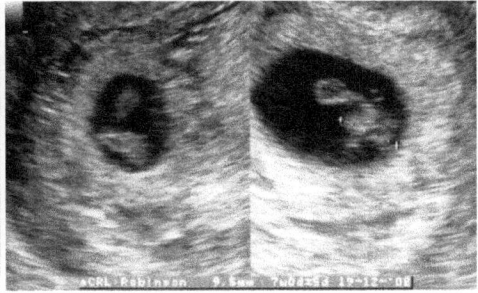

4.17b

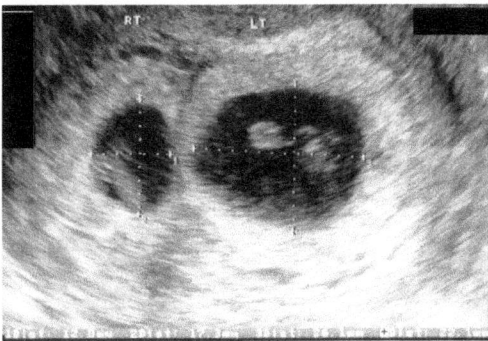

4.17c

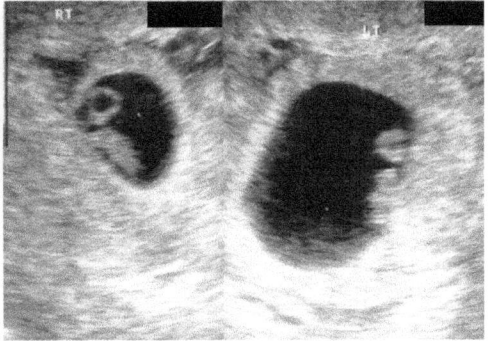

4.17d

Ultrasound findings: DC/DA twins (4.17a–d). The GS for the twin on the right is still smaller than the GS for twin on the left (4.17c–d). However, their CRLs are comparable (8.9mm and 9.5mm)(4.17a–b).

Impression: DC/DA twins with asymmetrical GS sizes.
* Throughout the pregnancy there was discrepancy in the GS sizes, but the sizes of the fetuses were comparable and the pregnancy was otherwise uneventful.

4.18

This patient was referred at 20+ 5 with a history of ? SROM

HC = 95mm = 13+6. Other fetal measurements were unobtainable.

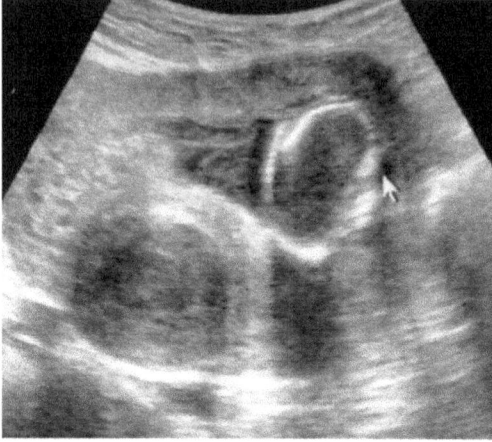

4.18a

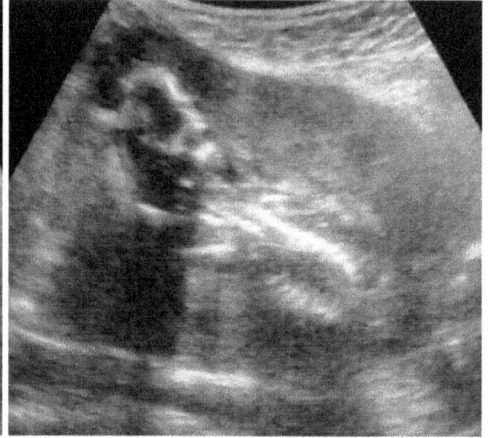

4.18b

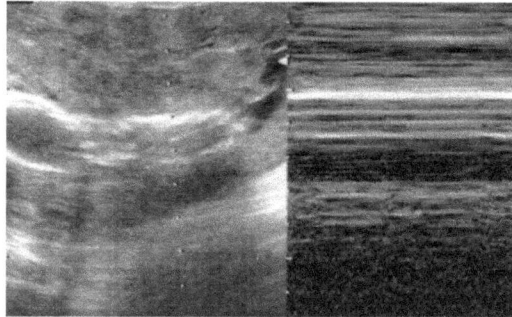

4.18c

Ultrasound findings: A single IU gestation with a fetus but no FHB (4.18c). The Spalding's sign in the fetal head indicates that fetal demise has been a while ago (4.18a). No amniotic fluid is demonstrated (4.18a–c). There is a posterior intramural fibroid (measurement has not been included 4.18a).

Impression: IUD

* Lack of amniotic fluid makes it difficult to assess fetal anatomy.

* Spalding's sign, i.e. overlapping of the cranial bones (see arrows above) is indicative of fetal demise. Spalding's sign is estimated to occur 4–7 days after fetal IUD.

4.19

This patient was referred at 11+3/40 by the GP with a history of positive pregnancy test result and maternal anxiety.

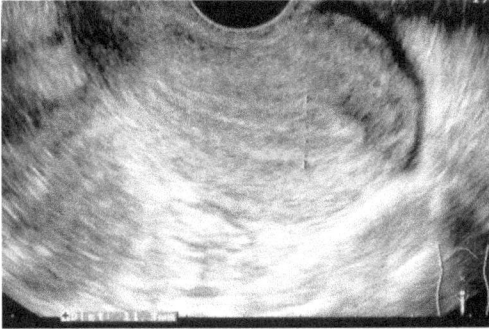
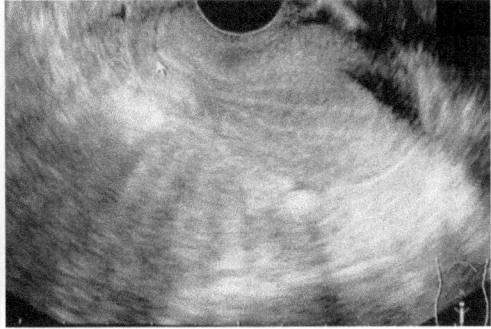

| 4.19a | 4.19b |

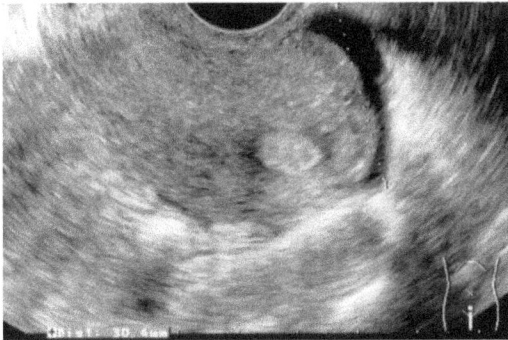
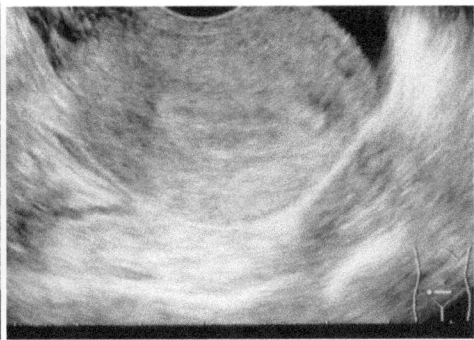

| 4.19c | 4.19d |

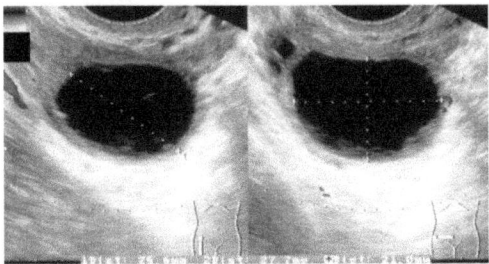
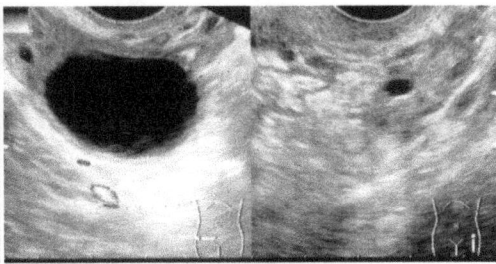

| 4.19e | 4.19f |

Ultrasound findings: A retroverted uterus with an 11mm triple line endometrium. There is tiny fluid in the cervical canal (4.19b arrow head) and around the uterine fundus up to 30mm in depth (4.19a–d). The left ovary appears normal (4.19f second half) and in the right ovary is a 26 × 28 × 21mm corpus luteum (4.19e).

Impression: No obvious IUGS is demonstrated rather ultrasound appearances are suggestive of recent ovulation. Suggest repeat pregnancy test.

* In-house pregnancy test result after the scan was negative.

4.20

This patient was referred with a history of ?SROM and infection at 16+5/40. Not shown here is AC=105mm=16+2/40. BDP = 31mm=15+1/40

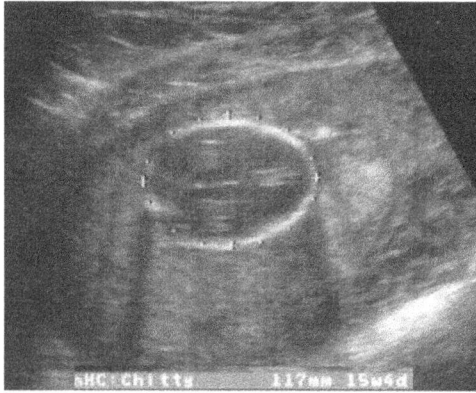

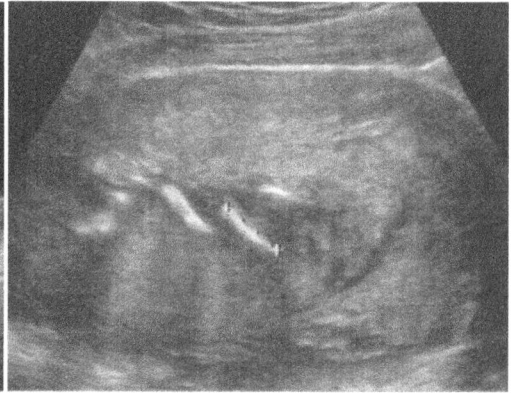

4.20a   *4.20b*

++17mm = 14+6/40

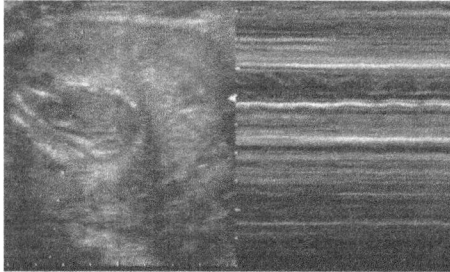

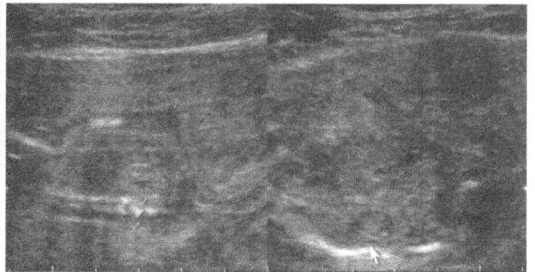

4.20c.   *4.20d.*

Arrows pointing to the kidneys

Ultrasound findings: Singleton pregnancy with FHB (4.20c). Both kidneys and urinary bladder are noted (4.20d). Anhydramnios (4.20a–b).

Fetal measurements – BPD = 31mm = 15+2,

HC = 117 = 15+4, AC = 105mm =16+2,

FL = 17mm = 14+6.

Impression: Single intrauterine pregnancy with FHB. Renal agenesis has been excluded as the cause of the anhydramnios. Should the pregnancy continue, the fetus is susceptible to lung hypoplasia and limb deformity.

* The prognosis of the pregnancy is not good.

* The patient unfortunately later miscarried.

Causes of anhydramnios include the following:

- Preterm premature rupture of membrane (PPROM)
- Fetal renal tract abnormality, e.g. agenesis
- Early onset of IUGR
- Placental insufficiency
- Silent uterine rupture
- Chemotherapeutic agents administered in pregnancy

4.21

This patient was referred with a history of 20/7 pv. bleeding and maternal anxiety at 7+0/40. Previous two miscarriages.

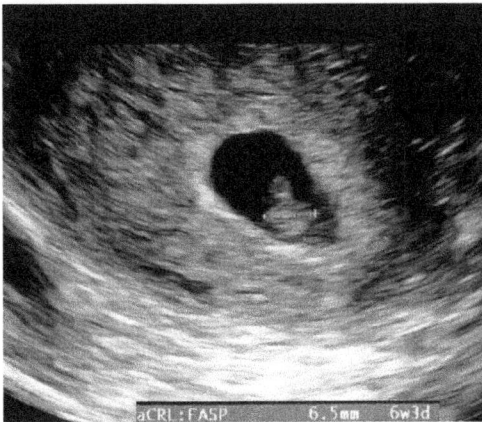
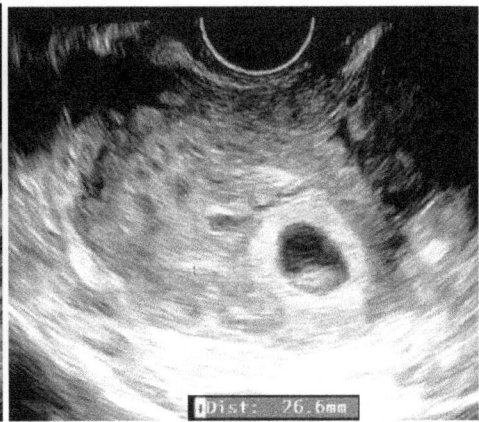

4.21a	**4.21b**

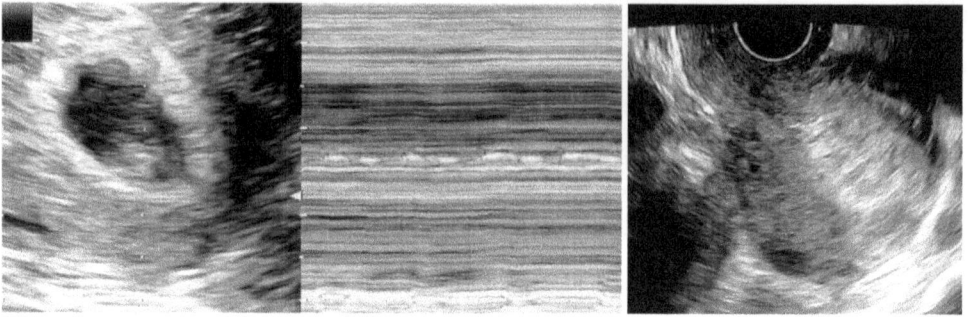

4.21c

4.21d

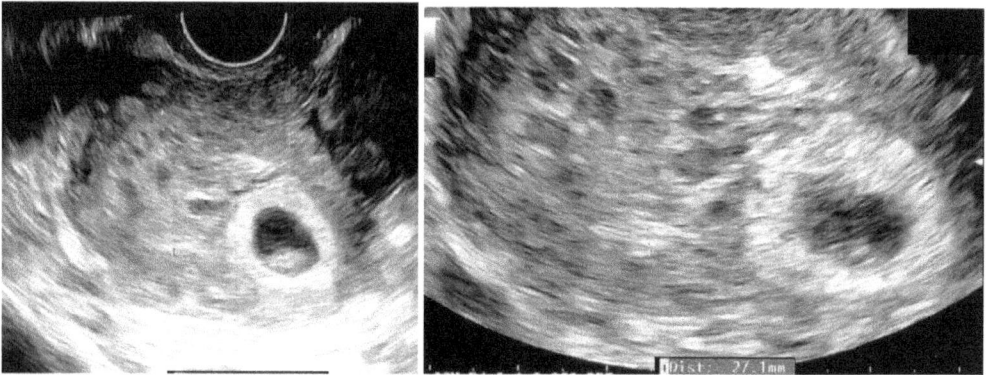

4.21e

4.21f

Ultrasound findings: Septate uterus with singleton pregnancy in the left horn (4.21b, e–f,). Embryonic pole, EHR (4.21a–d), CRL = 6.5mm = 6+1/40 (4.21a). Endometrial thickness on the right is 26mm and cystic in appearance (4.21b, d-f).

Impression: Septate uterus with singleton pregnancy in the left horn. Decidual reaction in the right endometrium which is likely to be the cause of the long-standing pv. bleed.

4.22

This patient was referred with a history of anxiety and pain.

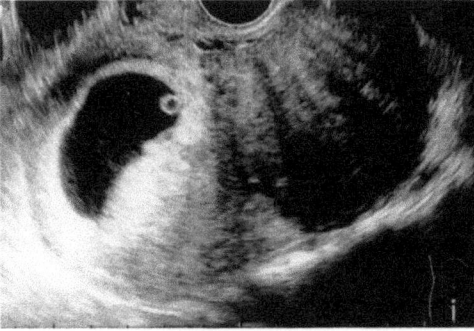
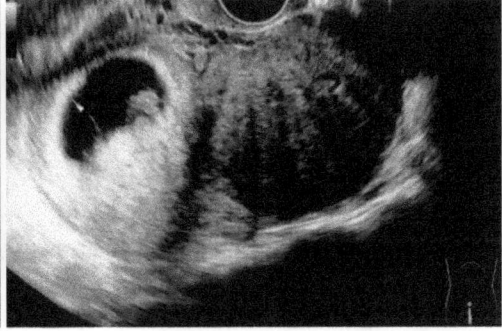

4.22a   **4.22b**

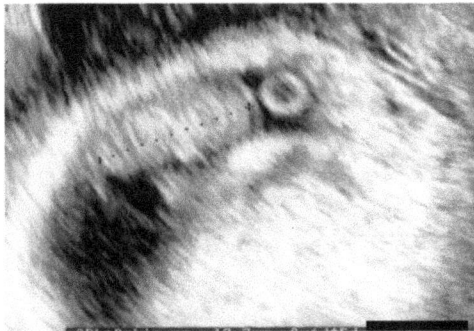
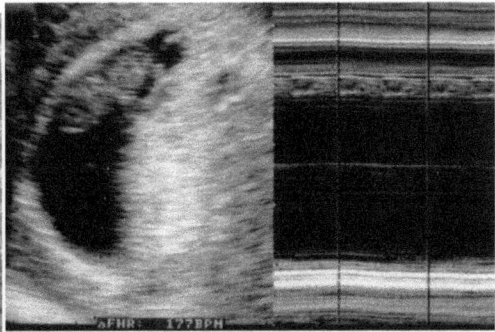

4.22c   **4.22d**

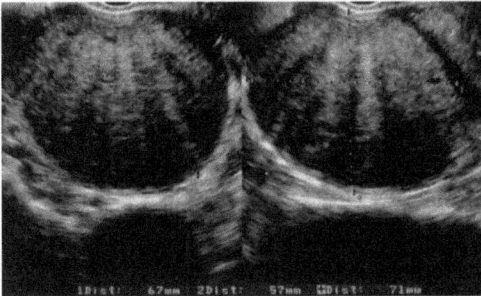
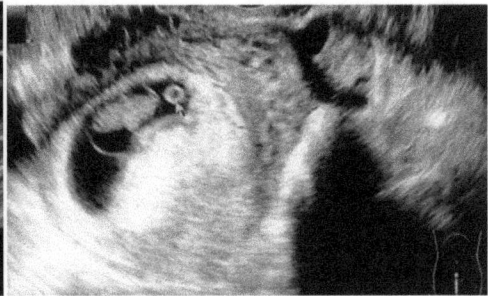

4.22e   **4.22f**

Ultrasound findings: Singleton pregnancy and in the posterior cervix is an approx. 67 × 57 × 71mm fibroid (4.22e). There is an embryo, yolk sac. (4.22a–e and f), embryonic pole, EHR (4.22d), CRL = 18.7mm = 8+4/40 (4.22c).

Impression: Singleton ongoing pregnancy. Cervical fibroid is noted.

4.23

This patient was referred for a scan with a history of uncertain dates as she conceived whilst breastfeeding. Left ovary was not visualised. There was a small CLC in the right ovary (not shown below).

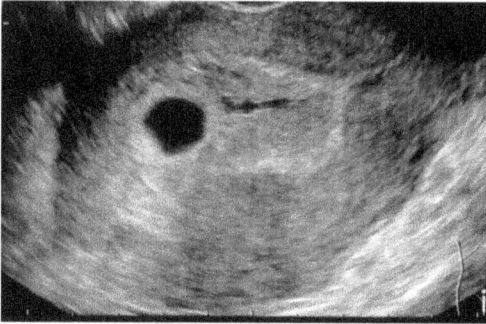

4.23a

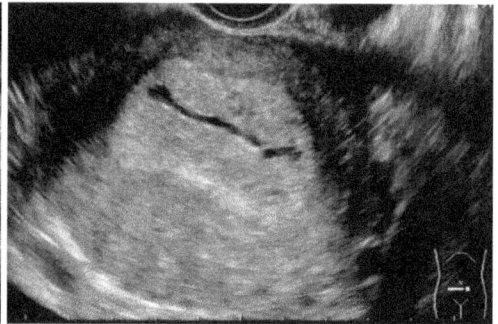

4.23b

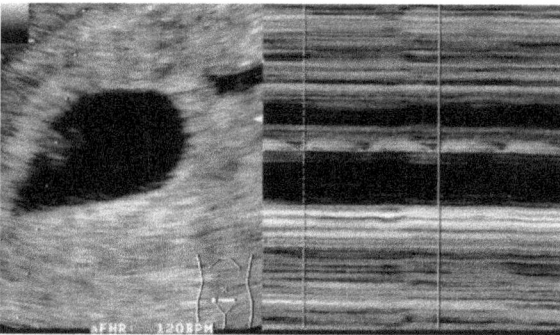

4.23c

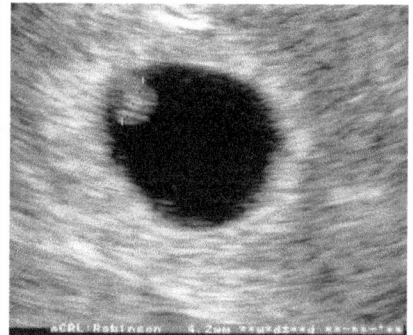

4.23d

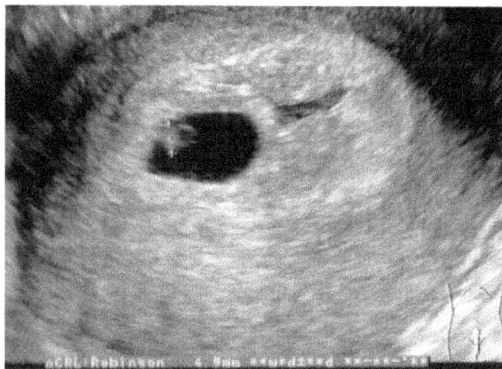

4.23e

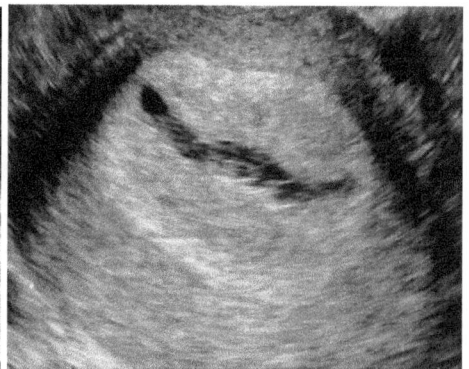

4.23f

Ultrasound findings: An IUGS, YS, FP (423.a, c, d) and EHB is seen. (4.23c) 120bpm. CRL = 4.9mm. Superior and to the left of the GS is a small area of bleeding (422.e–f). Follow-up scan will depend on the departmental protocol.

Impression: Single IUP with an area of bleeding to the left of the GS.

4.24

This patient was referred with a history of pv. bleeding.

Both ovaries (not shown here) appeared sonographically normal.

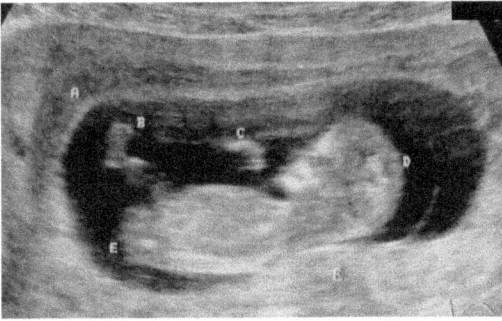

4.24a

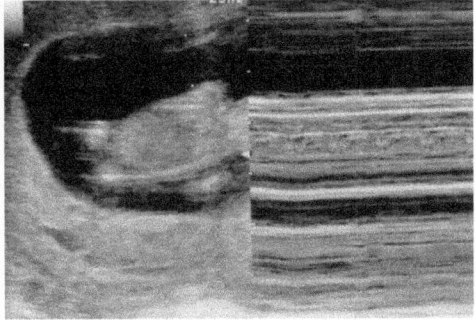

4.24b

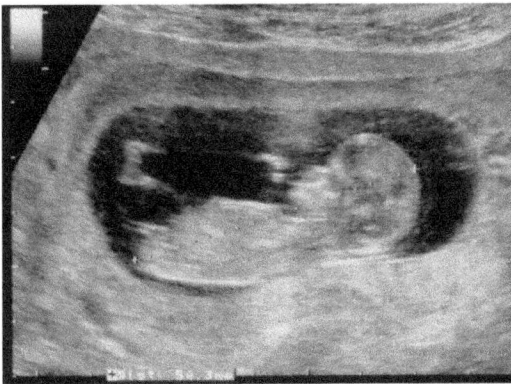

4.24c

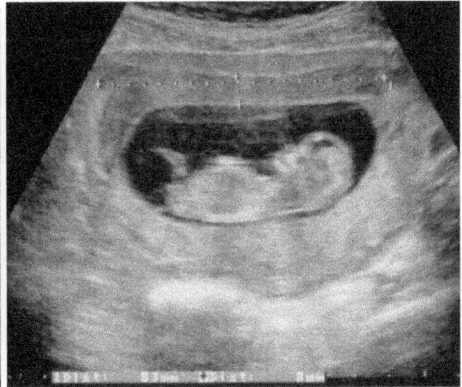

4.24d

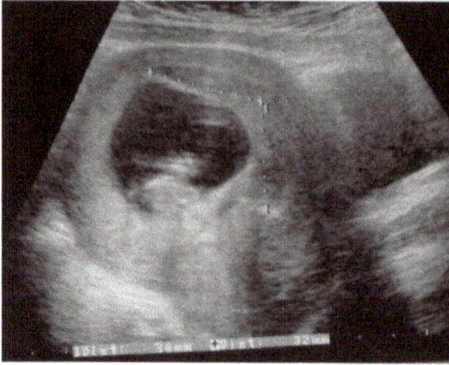
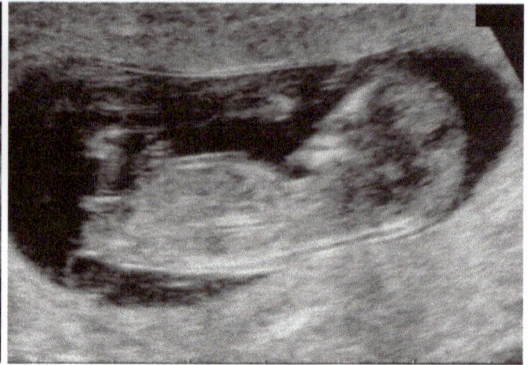

| 4.24e | 4.24f |

Note the rump/bottom superior to the YS in 4.24f.

A – Area of bleed, B – foot, C – hand, D – head/crown,

E – rump or bottom, F – posterior placenta. (4.23a)

Ultrasound findings: Single IUGS, fetus, yolk sac and FHB seen (4.24a–d, d, f). CRL = 54.3mm (4.24c). Superior and lateral to the GS, is an approx. 34 × 83 × 8mm hypoechoic area (4.24c–e).

Impression: Single IUGS and fetus with FHB. Superior and lateral to the GS is a hypoechoic area. This is likely to be a haematoma/bleed.

4.25

This patient was initially referred for a scan with a history of pv. bleeding.

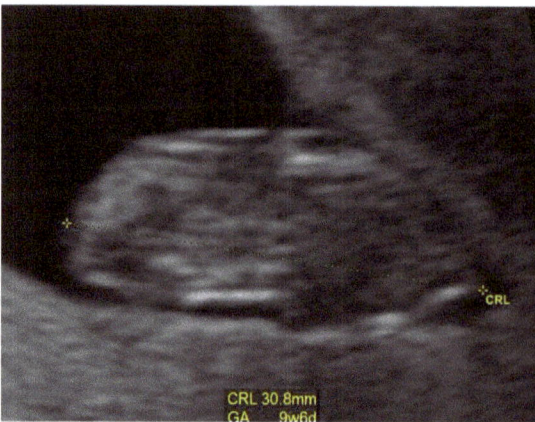
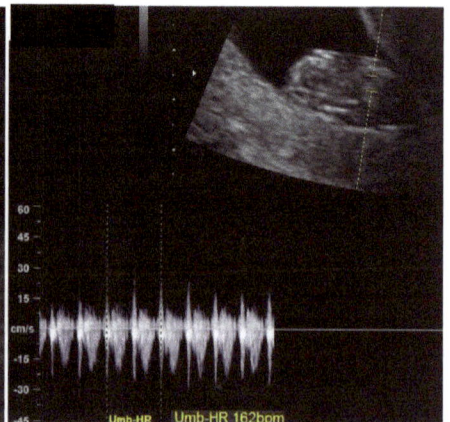

| 4.25a | 4.25b |

Two weeks later:

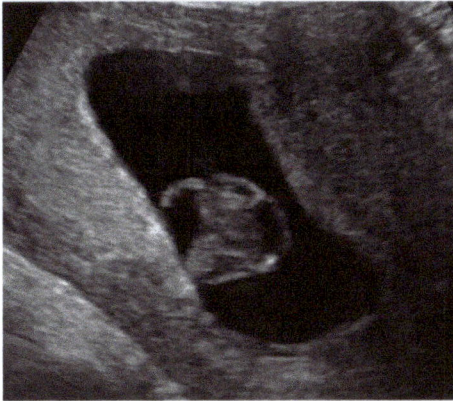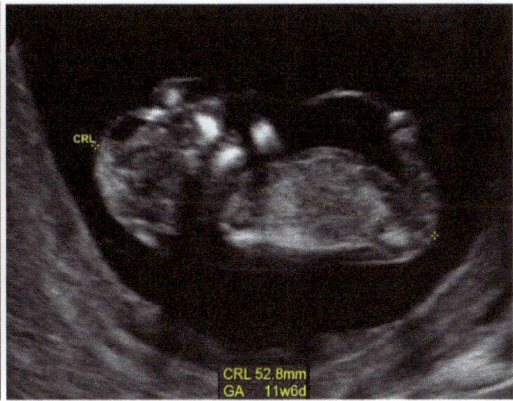

4.25c   **4.25d**

Ultrasound findings: Singleton pregnancy with FHB. CRL = 30.8mm = 9+6/40. FHB= 162bpm (4.25a–b).

Two weeks later: Singleton pregnancy. CRL = 52.8mm = 11+6/40 (4.25d) with abnormal brain appearance (4.25c–d). The fetal growth within the 2 weeks interval is normal.

Impression: abnormal brain and facial appearance.

* Follow-up scan confirmed ? facial cleft and early rupture of the membranes.

*This is not good news to tell the patient.

4.26

This patient was referred with a history of maternal anxiety. GA by LMP = 8+6/40.

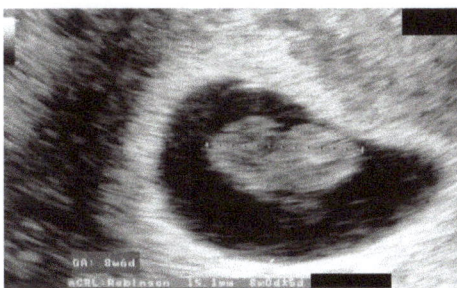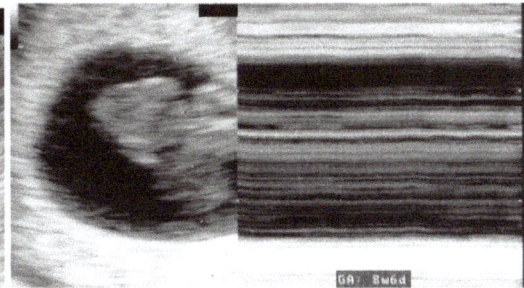

4.26a   **4.26b**

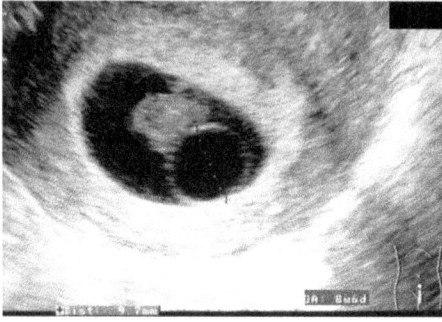 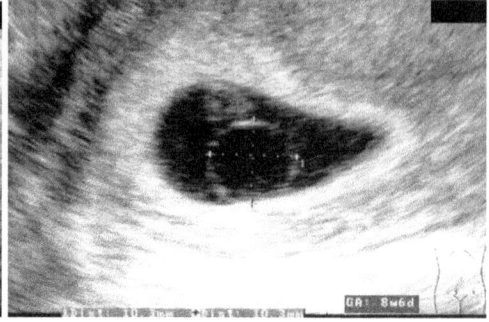

4.26c   **4.26d**

YS – 10.3 × 10.3 × 9.7mm

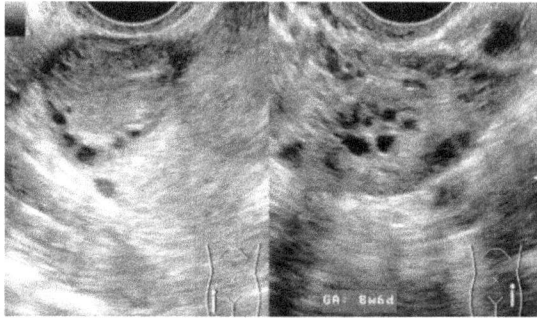

4.26e

Right ovarian volume = 11ml. Left ovarian volume *(not shown here)* = 9ml.

Ultrasound findings: An IUGS, YS, FP but no FHB (4.26a–b). CRL – 15.1mm = 8/40 (4.26a). GA by LMP = 8+6/40. There is an abnormally large yolk sac (4.26c–d), right PCO. Left ovary appear sonographically normal (4.26e).

Impression: Missed abortion or miscarriage.

4.27

This patient was referred with a history of abdominal pain at 5+4/40. Natural conception.

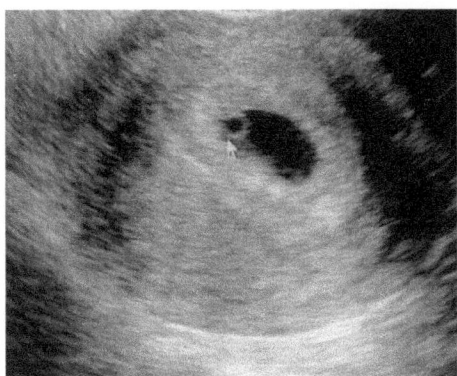 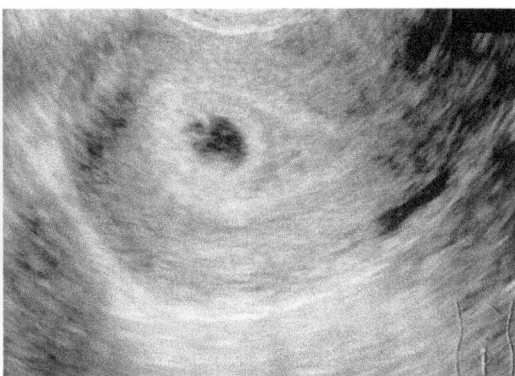

4.27a   4.27b

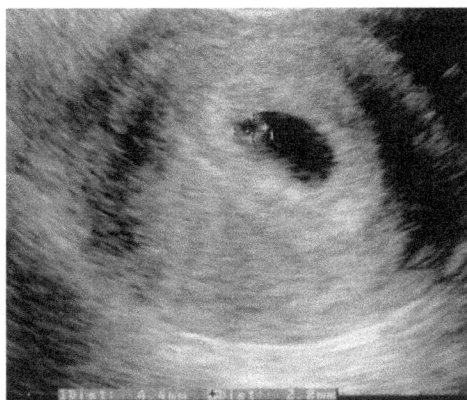 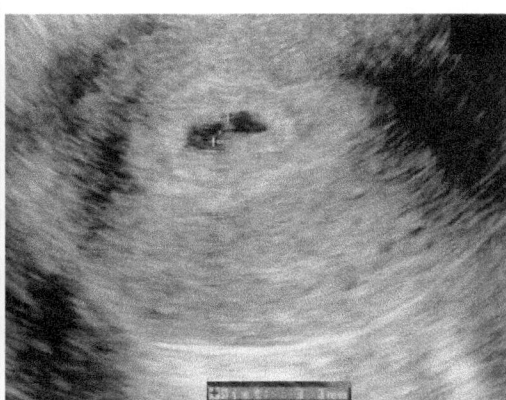

4.27c   4.27d

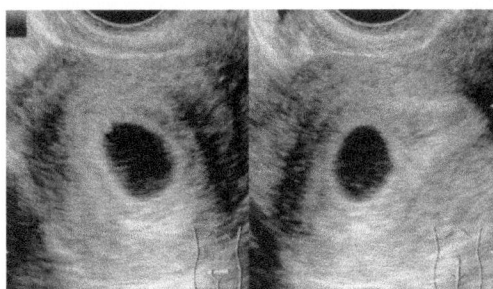 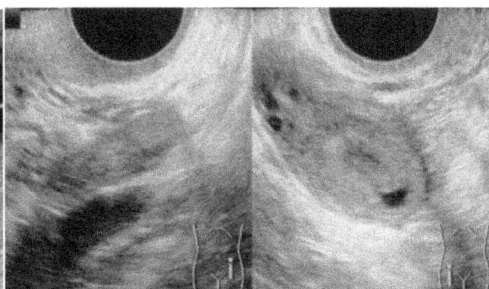

4.27e   4.27f

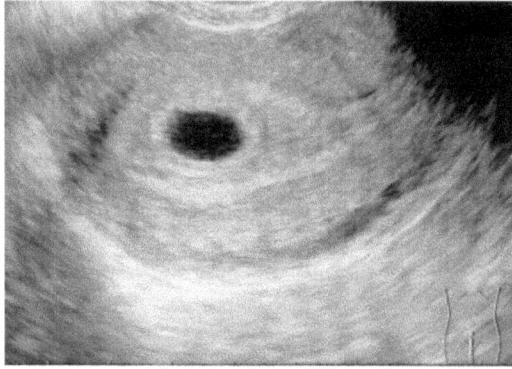

4.27g

Ultrasound findings: IUGS measuring and YS measuring 3 × 4 × 3mm (27a–e). There is a corpus luteum in the right ovary. Lt ovary appears sonographically normal (4.27f).

Impression: Early pregnancy – viability uncertain at this early GA. A follow-up scan should be arranged.

It is not unusual not to be able to find the ultrasound cause of abdominal pains. GIT and kidneys, ureters and bladder (KUB) problems will need to be excluded

4.28

This patient was referred for a scan with a history of light pv. bleeding for some days before the scan.

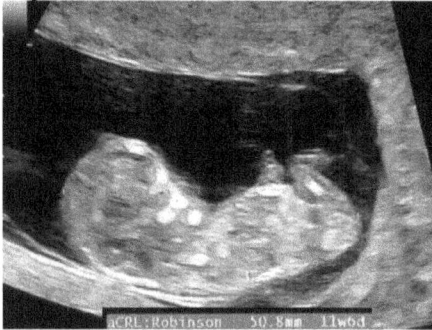
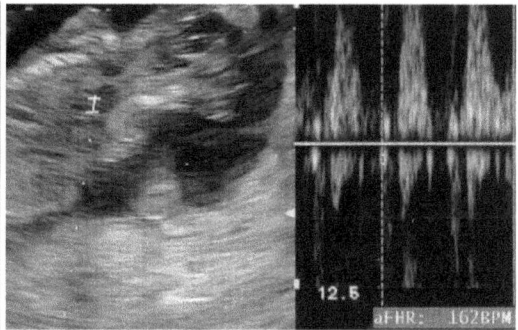

4.28a   **4.28b**

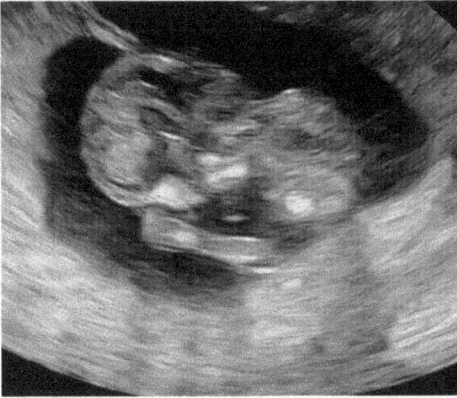

4.28c

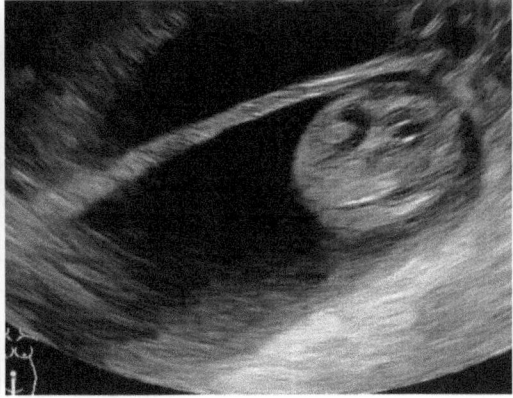

4.28d

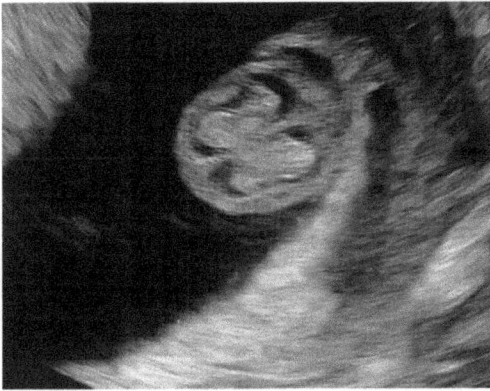

4.28e

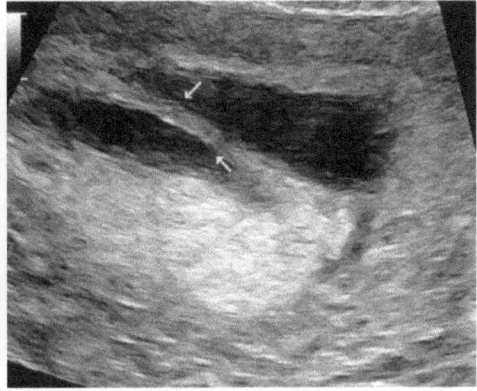

4.28f

Ultrasound findings: Singleton intrauterine pregnancy with FHB of 162bpm. CRL = 50.8mm =11+6/40 (4.28a–b). Stretching across the uterus is a thick band or sheet. No fetal part is demonstrated above as caught in it. Arrows in 4.28f (4.28c–f).

Impression: Singleton pregnancy with FHB. There is a uterine synechia present.

4.29

This patient was referred at 9+2/40 because of maternal anxiety and pvb. A CLC not shown here was seen in the left ovary. Right ovary not shown here appeared sonographically normal.

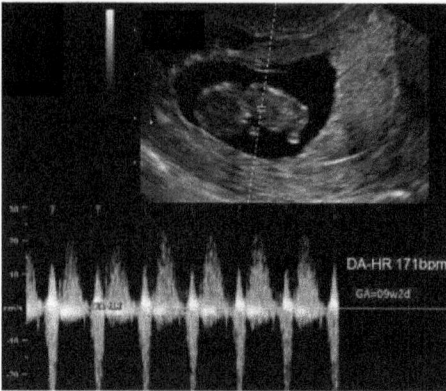

4.29a

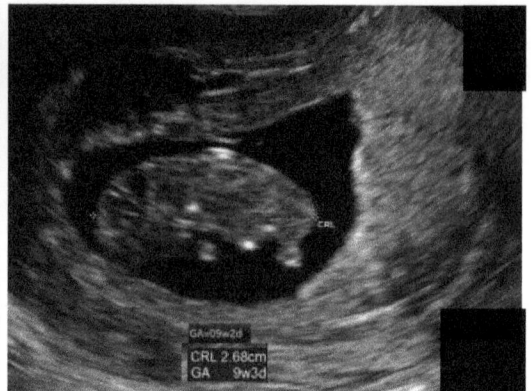

4.29b

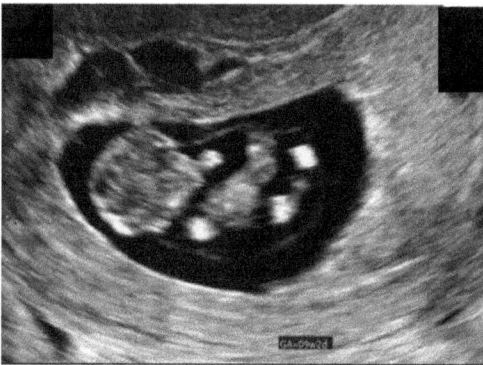

4.29c

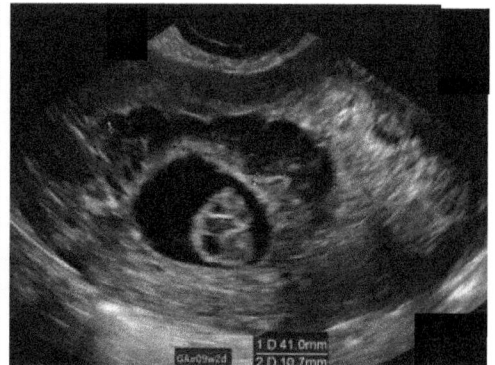

4.29d

Ultrasound findings: Single IUP. CRL = 26.8mm = 9+3/40. (4.29b) EHR = 171bpm. Superior to the gestational sac is an irregular in outline predominantly hypoechoic area measuring 41 x 11mm. This is most likely an area of bleed,

Impression: Single on going pregnancy with a 41 x 11mm probably implantational bleed

4.30

Shown here are the images of an ultrasound scan that was done at 12/40 by GA. Patient was very sure of her dates. Both ovaries (not shown here) appeared sonographically normal.

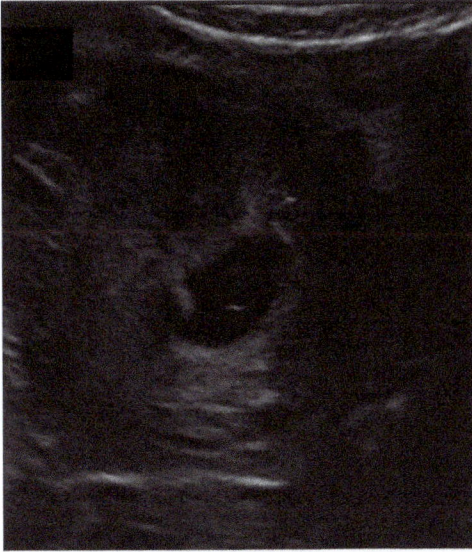

4.30a

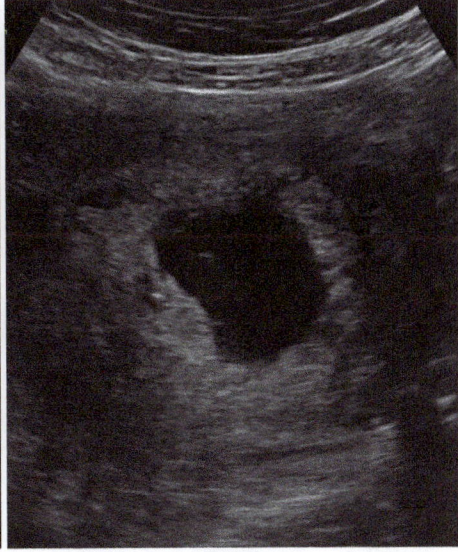

4.30b

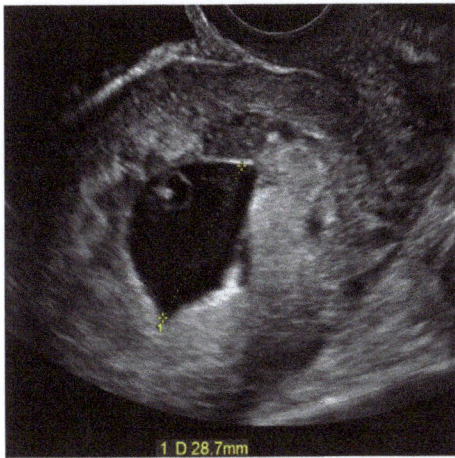

4.30c

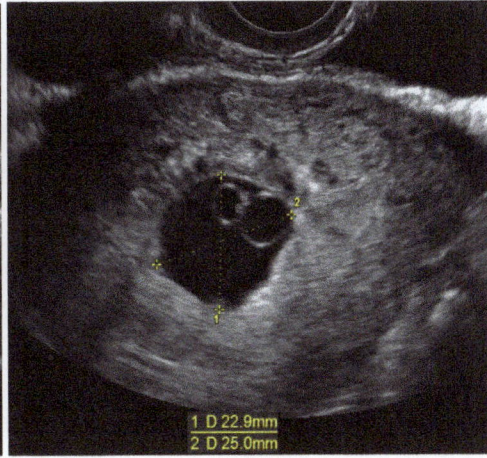

4.30d

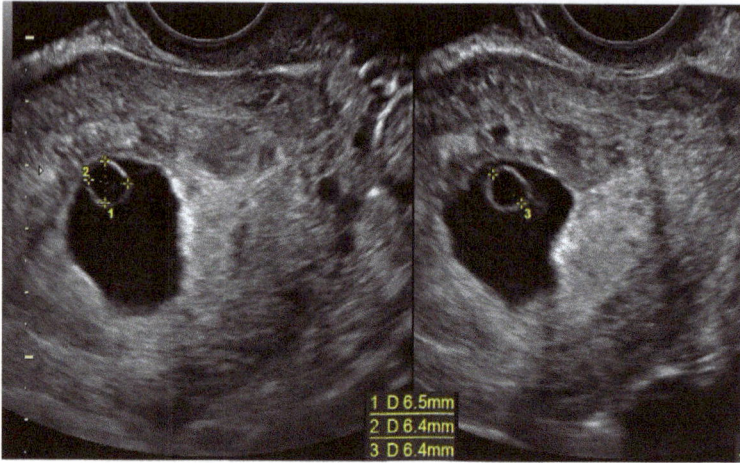

4.30e

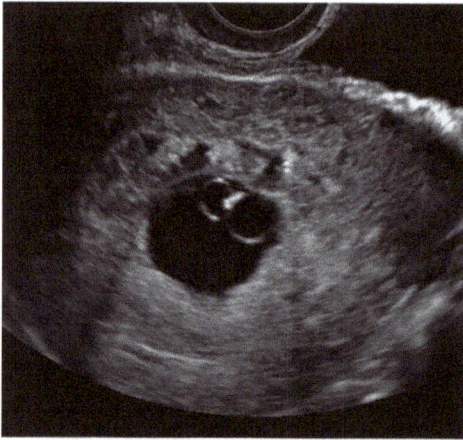

4.30f

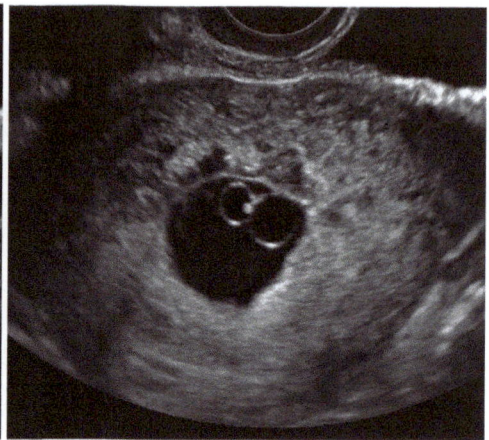

4.30g

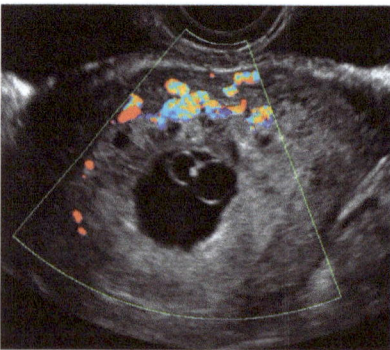

4.30h

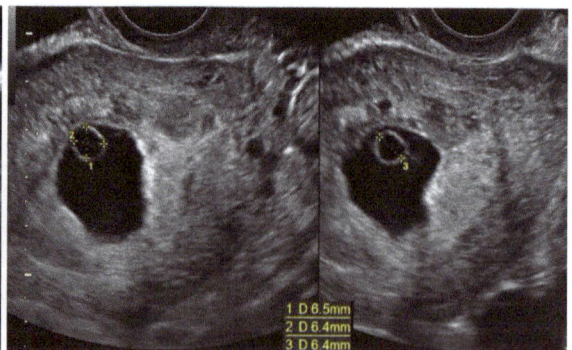

4.30i

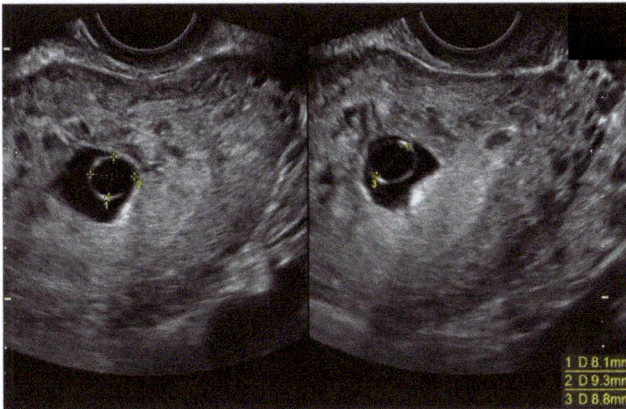

4.30j

Ultrasound findings: An irregularly shaped intrauterine GS measuring approx. 29 × 23 × 25mm (4.30c–d). In it are two cystic bubbles measuring approx. 6.5 × 6.4 × 6.4mm and 8.1 × 9.3 × 8.8 mm (30d–j).? double bleb sign.

Impression: Irregular in outline IUGS < than dates.

Patient subsequently miscarried.

Chapter Conclusion

Although women may present with similar clinical conditions, it is not unusual to find non-similar ultrasound appearances – some that may have uncomplicated features, others that may be complex.

In complex cases a good or clear description of what has been seen, including the relevant measurements will be ideal and can help clinicians to establish a diagnosis.

The role of the Sonographer in EPAGU includes: (in no particular order)

- Arriving at a diagnosis i.e. being able to answer the question or reason for the scan and where the diagnosis is not straight forward being able to describe the ultrasound appearances as clearly as possible.
- Reassuring the patient where possible e.g. a confirmed single intrauterine pregnancy cannot change and become an ectopic pregnancy subsequently.
- Educating the patient or relatives e.g. weekly scan cannot guarantee no miscarriage.
- Departmental protocols need to be adhered to in order to avoid unnecessary repeat scan examinations.
- Showing good quality care in communication and empathy.
- Be humble and comfortable to ask for a second opinion with the patient or couple's consent as some situations are 1 in many thousands.
- Be willing to learn from others - no one knows it all or have seen it all.
- Follow up interesting cases - it is a good way of learning and getting better.
- Attend MTD meetings when and where available.
- Using the appropriate obstetric graphs tend to make the ultrasound findings easier to understand and explain to the patient or couple.

As a Sonographer working in EPAGU be prepared to: .

- Perform TVS and interpret it.
- Communicate 'bad news' to the patient/couple
- Get a second opinion
- Be flexible in technique
- Refer to the Consultant

- Suggest further imaging where applicable
- Identify embryo or fetal abnormality relative to fetal GA
- Identify serious maternal problems e.g. complex ovarian cyst or mass.
- Have your own suitable way of dealing with work related stress especially that which is related to many times repeatedly having to give 'bad news' to patients.

Book Conclusion
(not in any particular order)

The Sonographer:
- Should have and exibit good communication skills
- Should be familiar with department protocols and policies
- Should be able to answer the question on the request form
- Should be comfortable with performing and interpreting TVS
- Should be humble enough to ask for a second opinion if need be
- Should be familiar with the normal ultrasound appearances of the embryo or fetal anatomy
- Should be familiar with the ultrasound appearances of a normal female pelvis
- Should be able to communicate nicely and clearly ultrasound findings that are 'bad news' to the patient or couple
- If possible he should be familiar with performing and interpreting 3D ultrasound where the facility is available
- Not every ultrasound finding is straight forward, when a diagnosis or impression is unclear, he should at least be able describe what he has seen during the ultrasound examination
- Having a good rapport with the other multidisciplinary team members in our experience makes the work easier
- Should attend relevant MTD meetings
- Should keep abreast of latest information and technique as this is essential for good quality practice
- Working in EPAGU for the Sonographer could be challenging, keeping calm under pressure and following one's routine pattern of scanning will help in not missing pathology or abnormalities
- Workflow could be heavy, busy and demanding but don't neglect your health - stretch regularly during the session, hydrate yourself and find time to visit the toilet if need be
- Avoid RSI

Appendix 1

Obstetric graphs

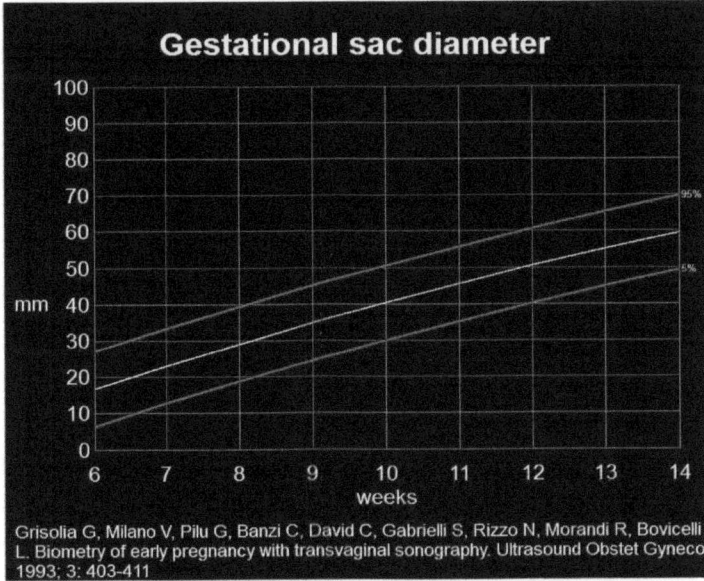

Gestational sac diameter

Grisolia G, Milano V, Pilu G, Banzi C, David C, Gabrielli S, Rizzo N, Morandi R, Bovicelli L. Biometry of early pregnancy with transvaginal sonography. Ultrasound Obstet Gynecol 1993; 3: 403-411

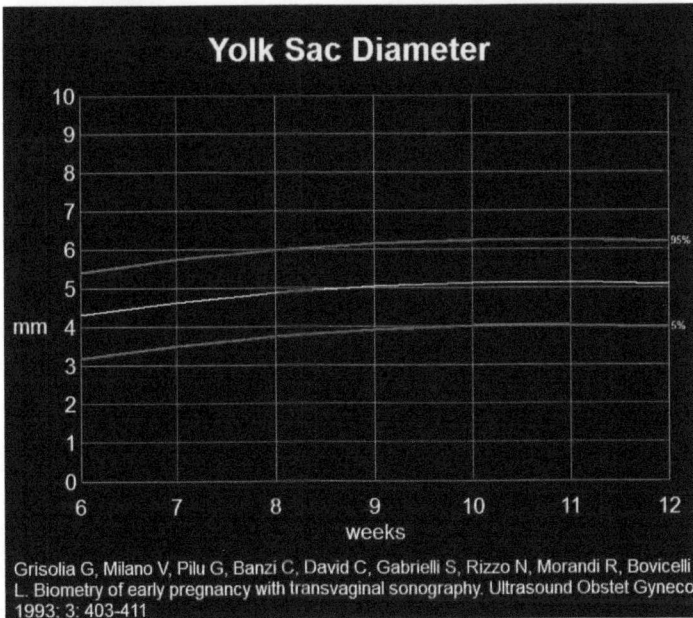

Yolk Sac Diameter

Grisolia G, Milano V, Pilu G, Banzi C, David C, Gabrielli S, Rizzo N, Morandi R, Bovicelli L. Biometry of early pregnancy with transvaginal sonography. Ultrasound Obstet Gynecol 1993; 3: 403-411

Crown-rump length

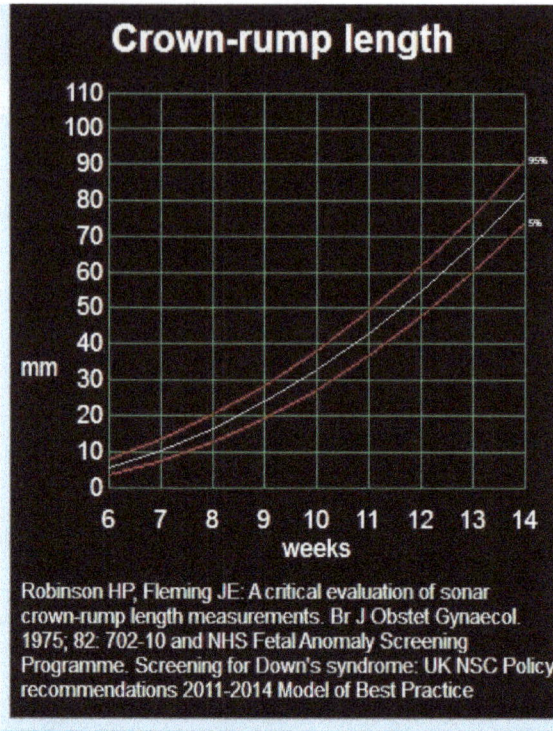

Robinson HP, Fleming JE: A critical evaluation of sonar crown-rump length measurements. Br J Obstet Gynaecol. 1975; 82: 702-10 and NHS Fetal Anomaly Screening Programme. Screening for Down's syndrome: UK NSC Policy recommendations 2011-2014 Model of Best Practice

Fetal heart rate

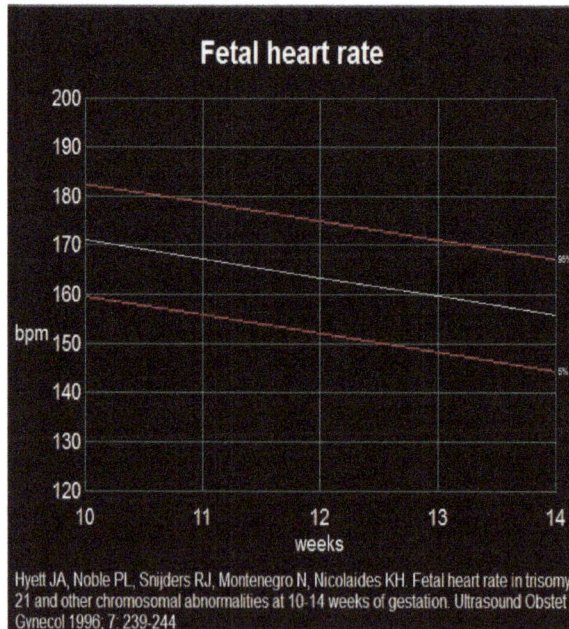

Hyett JA, Noble PL, Snijders RJ, Montenegro N, Nicolaides KH. Fetal heart rate in trisomy 21 and other chromosomal abnormalities at 10-14 weeks of gestation. Ultrasound Obstet Gynecol 1996; 7: 239-244

Biparietal diameter

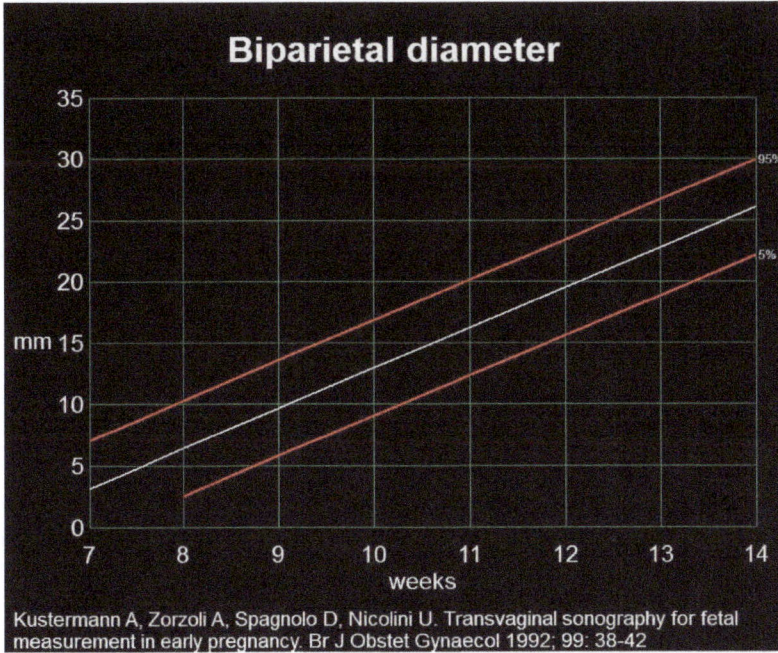

Kustermann A, Zorzoli A, Spagnolo D, Nicolini U. Transvaginal sonography for fetal measurement in early pregnancy. Br J Obstet Gynaecol 1992; 99: 38-42

Head circumference

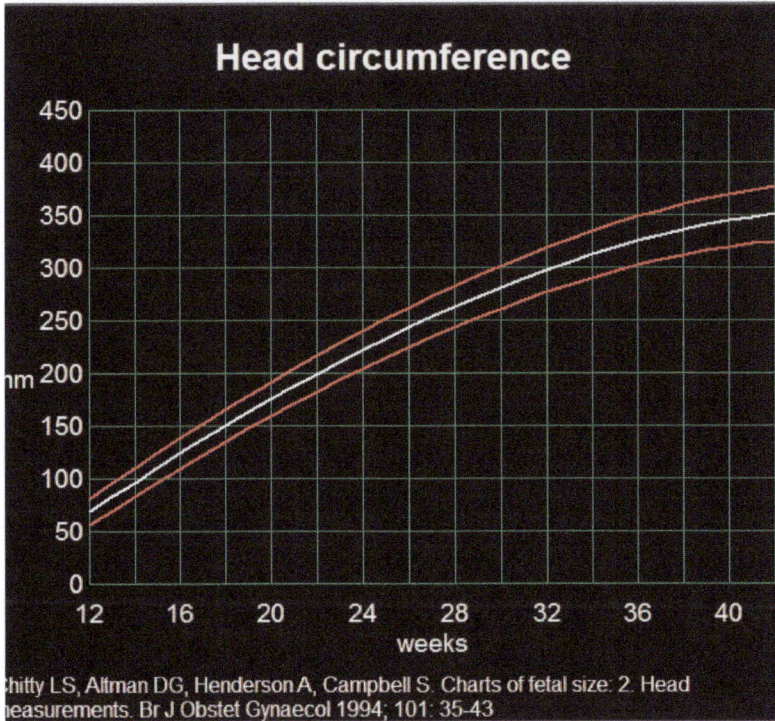

Chitty LS, Altman DG, Henderson A, Campbell S. Charts of fetal size: 2. Head measurements. Br J Obstet Gynaecol 1994; 101: 35-43

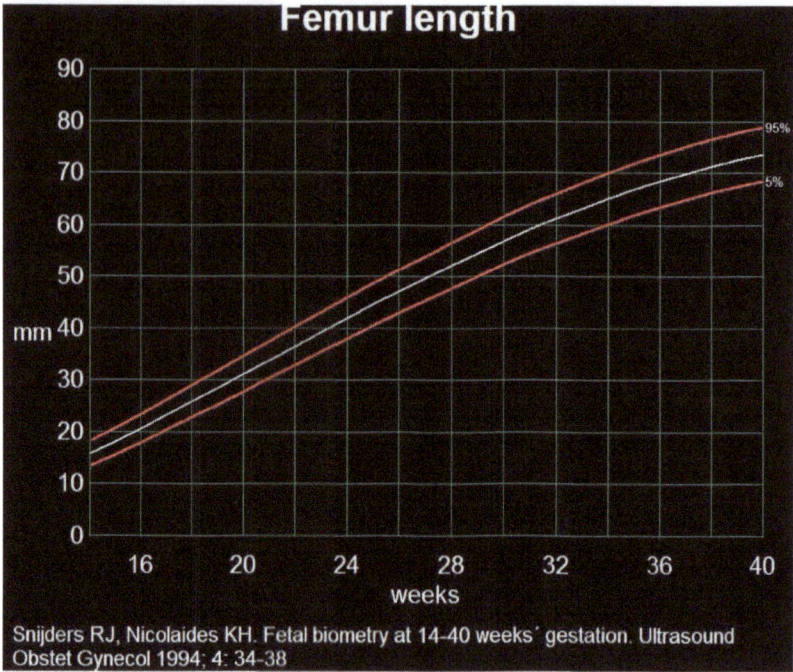

Femur length

Snijders RJ, Nicolaides KH. Fetal biometry at 14-40 weeks' gestation. Ultrasound Obstet Gynecol 1994; 4: 34-38

As the AC is not used for dating a pregnancy, the AC graph has not been included in this section.

Appendix 2

An example of an ultrasound examination request form that could be used in EPAGU.

- Hospital/GP details:
- Patient's details:

• Surname:	• LMP:
• First Name:	• Menstrual Cycle: regular / Irregular
• Date of Birth:	• Average length of Cycle: days
• Hospital Number:	• Pregnancy test result: Positive/Negative
• View Point Number if known:	• ß-HCG level if known:

- Reason for today's scan. Please tick or circle all that applies.
- Bleeding: Yes ☐   No ☐
- Spotting ☐ Light bleeding ☐ Heavy bleeding ☐ Since when (date)?
- Abdominal/Pelvic pains: Yes ☐ No Localised ☐ Generalised ☐
- Since when date?
- Nausea ☐ Vomiting ☐ Hyperemesis ☐
- Missing IUCD: Which type: Mirena ☐ Copper T ☐ No idea ☐
- ? Ectopic:
- Maternal anxiety
- Post-miscarriage:
- Previous miscarriage
- Conceived on the pill
- Recommended follow-up
- Unknown or unsure of LMP
- Conceived with the coil in situ
- Post-fertility treatment: Yes ☐ No ☐
- Which type: Clomid ☐ Metformin ☐ IUI ☐ IVF ☐ ICSI ☐ SUZI ☐
- How many embryos were transferred?
- What date was the embryo transfer done?
- Other reasons and relevant history. Please specify:
- Referring clinician & Designation: Date:--/--/--

Further Reading

The following publications are recommended as source reading for most aspects of obstetrics and gynaecology ultrasound. Books and articles relating to more specific aspects are listed under the individual chapters:

Books

Andrews H. (2001) Ultrasound in Obstetrics & Gynaecology. KC. Dewbury KC [et al.] (editors). London. Churchill Livingstone.

Bates J. (editor) (1997) Practical Gynaecological Ultrasound. London. Greenwich Medical Media Ltd.

Bates J. (editor) (2006) Practical Gynaecological Ultrasound. 2nd ed. London. Greenwich Medical Media Ltd.

Benson CB, Bluth EI. (editors) (2008) Ultrasonography in Obstetrics and Gynaecology: A Practical Approach to Clinical problems. 2nd ed. Stuttgart, Germany. Thieme.

Chudleigh P, Thilaganathan B. (2004) Obstetric Ultrasound: How, Why and When. 3rd ed. Edinburgh, New York. Elsevier Churchill Livingstone.

Ola-Ojo O. O. (2005) Obstetrics and Gynaecology Ultrasound: A Self-Assessment Guide. Edinburgh, New York. Elsevier Churchill Livingstone.

Sanders RC. (1991) Clinical Ultrasonography – A Practical Guide. 2nd ed. Boston, USA. Little, Brown.

eBook

Abuhamad A. (editor) (2014) Ultrasound in Obstetrics and Gynaecology – A practical approach, eBook, Contributions from Chaoui Rabih, Jeanty Philippe, Paladini Dario.

Articles

Board of the Faculty of Clinical Radiology. The Royal College of Radiologists, Council; the Royal College of Obstetricians and Gynaecologists. Guidance on Ultrasound Procedures in Early Pregnancy (1995) RCR Ref Number BFCR(95)B. ISBN: 1872599168.

Guidelines for Professional Working Standards: Ultrasound Practice (2008) Society of Radiographers. London. http://www.sor.org/learning/do cument-library/guidelines-professional-working-standards-ultrasound-practice

Useful websites and addresses

American Institute of Ultrasound in Medicine: http://www.aium.org

The American Institute of Ultrasound in Medicine (AIUM) is a multidisciplinary organisation dedicated to advancing the art and science of ultrasound in medicine and research through its educational, scientific, literary and professional activities. The website contains a useful menu selection on Standards for the Performance of Ultrasound Examination.

British Medical Ultrasound Society

36 Portland Place

London W1B 1LS

Tel: 020 7636 3914

http://www.bmus.org

The British Medical Ultrasound Society (BMUS) includes amongst its aims the advancement of the science and technology of ultrasonics as applied to medicine, as well as the provision of advice and information regarding ultrasound to the general public. It also provides links to affiliated societies concerned with the science and application of ultrasound.

The Ectopic Pregnancy Trust,

3rd floor

28 Portland Place

London

W1B 1LY

http://www.ectopic.org.uk

Tel: 020 7733 2653

Supporting people who have experienced an early pregnancy complication and the healthcare professionals who care for them

European Federation of Societies for Ultrasound in Medicine and Biology:

http://www.efsumb.org

The Federation's (EFSUMB) purpose is to promote the exchange of scientific knowledge and development in the medical and biological professions as applied to ultrasound, proposing standards and giving advice concerning criteria for the optimum apparatus and techniques together with presentation and interpretation of results.

http://www.jultrasoundmed.org:
The Journal of Ultrasound in Medicine (JUM) is dedicated to the rapid, accurate publication of original articles dealing with all aspects of medical ultrasound, particularly its direct application to patient care but also relevant to basic science, advances in instrumentation, and biological effects. The journal is an official publication of the American Institute of Ultrasound in Medicine and publishes articles in a variety of categories, including original research papers, review articles, pictorial essays, technical innovations, case series, letters to the editor, and more, from an international bevy of countries in a continual effort to showcase and promote advances in the ultrasound community.

http://209.217.125.17/SOGCnet/sogc docs/common/guide/pdfs/ps30.pdf
This website links the guidelines for the Performance of Ultrasound Examination in obstetrics and gynaecology with the policy statement document prepared by the Diagnostic Imaging Committee of the Society of Obstetricians and Gynaecologists of Canada. It outlines a standard for practitioners performing ultrasound studies of the female pelvis, including routine obstetrical ultrasound, fetal sex determination and use of ultrasound in delivery room emergencies.

Human Fertilisation & Embryology Authority
Paxton House
30 Artillery Lane
London E1 7LS
Tel: 0207 377 5077
http:www.hfea.gov.uk

The Human Fertilisation and Embryology Authority (HFEA), which was set up in the UK in 1991, ensures that all UK treatment clinics offering in vitro fertilisation (IVF) or donor insemination (DI), or storing eggs, sperm or embryos, conform to high medical and professional standards and are inspected regularly. They collect comprehensive data about such treatments, and provide detailed advice and information to the public. The publications section offers links to patient guides, code of practice and information leaflets.

International Federation of Gynecology and Obstetrics (FIGO) is a worldwide organisation of obstetricians and gynaecologists. The aims of FIGO are to promote the well-being of women and to raise the standard of practice in obstetrics and gynaecology. The website provides information about FIGO's activities, events and projects together with access to some of its publications including the FIGO newsletter, ethical guidelines and annual reports. http://www.figo.org/

The Miscarriage Association,
c/o Clayton Hospital
Northgate
Wakefield
West Yorkshire WF1 3JS
Tel (helpline): 01924 200799; admin: 01924 200795
Scottish helpline: 0131 334 8883 (answerphone with names of local contacts)
http://www.miscarriageassociation.org.uk
The Miscarriage Association publishes leaflets, fact sheets and audiotapes and has online information about miscarriage, ectopic pregnancy and molar pregnancy, including what is currently known about possible causes and the different treatments available. The association can provide information on the hospital provision of specialist services relating to pregnancy loss and it maintains a directory of other organisations which may also be of help.

Organising Medical Networked Information (OMNI) and Nursing, Midwifery and the Allied Health Professions (NMAP) are gateways to internet resources in medicine, biomedicine, allied health, health management and the Social Sciences. They aim to provide comprehensive coverage of the UK resources in both areas and provide access to the best resources worldwide.
http://www.omni.ac.uk and http://nmap.ac.uk/

Radiopaedia.org
The site provides a free educational radiology resource with one of the web's largest collections of radiology cases and reference articles. The site is targeted at

medical and radiology professionals, and contains user contributed content and material that may be confusing to a lay audience.

Royal College of Midwives
15 Mansfield Street
London W1G 9NH
Tel: 020 7312 3538
http://www.rcm.org.uk/
The Royal College of Midwives (RCM) is the only trade union and professional organisation run by midwives for midwives. It is the voice of midwifery, providing excellence in professional leadership, education, influence and representation for and on behalf of midwives. The RCM produces information and advice on a wide range of midwifery issues.

Royal College of Obstetricians and Gynaecologists
27 Sussex Place
Regents Park
London NW1 4RG
Tel: 020 7772 6309
http://www.rcog.org.uk/
The Royal College of Obstetricians and Gynaecologists (RCOG) states that its objectives are the encouragement of the study and the advancement of the science and practice of gynaecology. The RCOG publishes a number of guidelines on the use of ultrasound in its website Information Services section.

The Society and the College of Radiographers,
207 Providence Square
Mill Street
London SE1 2EW
Tel: 020 7740 7200
Fax: 020 7740 7205
http://www.sor.org.news.news.htm
The Society of Radiographers includes in its objectives the promotion and development of the science and practice of radiography and radiotherapeutic technology and allied subjects. It publishes the results of study and research work

therein and encourages public education, and it protects the honour and interests of those working in this field.

Sonoworld

http://sonoworld.com

A website that is dedicated to training and equipping professionals in ultrasound worldwide.

United Kingdom Association of Sonographers

36 Portland Place

London W1B 1LS

Tel: 0207 636 3714

http://www.ukasonographers.org

The United Kingdom Association of Sonographers (UKAS) produces guidelines that cover many areas, including medicolegal issues, audit and quality assurance, reporting of examinations, scanning procedures, communication to the patient and relevant clinician, ultrasound equipment usage and safe use and safety of ultrasound examination.

Wikipedia

Wikipedia is hosted by the Wikimedia Foundation, a non-profit organisation that also hosts a range of other projects. They provide free information on various subjects including medical conditions.

https://www.wikipedia.org

World Federation of Ultrasound in Medicine and Biology:

http://www.wfumb.org

World Federation of Ultrasound in Medicine and Biology (WFUMB) is a federation of affiliated organisations consisting of regional federations and national societies for ultrasound in medicine and biology, including the AIUM and EFSUMB mentioned above. WFUMB organises world congresses in ultrasound every 3 years covering the whole field of diagnostic ultrasound; it also organises and sponsors workshops on safety of ultrasound in medicine. Reports are published (monthly by Elsevier Science Inc.) in the official journal of WFUMB, Ultrasound in Medicine and Biology (UMB). See also www.elsevier.com/locate/ultrasmedbio

Other Ultrasound books by the Author

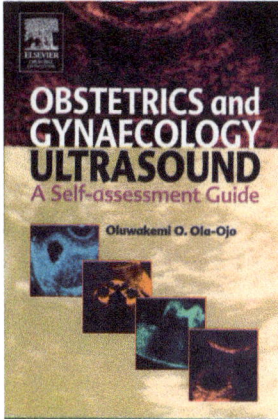

Obstetrics and Gynaecology Ultrasound - A Self-Assessment Guide
June 2005 Churchill Elsevier Publishers, UK.

This self-assessment guide is a structured questions and answer book that develops the reader's understanding capability using a simple method in treating related topics. Clinical indications are presented with their corresponding ultrasound findings using appropriate illustrations. A case study approach is followed; presenting the clinical and ethical dilemmas that might arise whilst encouraging students to think. The aim is to reinforce theoretical knowledge within a clinical environment.

Key features:
◆ Over 600 high-resolution ultrasound images
◆ Cover a wide spectrum of ultrasound curriculum.
◆ Includes a detailed study of fertility.
◆ Aids quick understanding of subject matter.
◆ 468 pages.

ISBN-10: 0443064628
ISBN-13: 978-0443064623

Book Dimensions: 24 x 16.8 x 2.6 cm
"...This excellent new book is a study guide... This is an attractive paperback that should be essential reading for trainee obstetric and gynaecological sonographers, whether they are radiographers or radiology or obstetric trainees. It will be of particular value to those preparing for the RCOG/RCR Diploma in Advanced Obstetric Ultrasound and to specialist registrars in obstetrics and gynaecology undertaking special skills modules in fetal medicine, gynaecological ultrasound and infertility..."

The Obstetrician & Gynaecologist, www.rcog.org.uk/togonline
Book reviews 2006

Reviewer **Ann Harper MD FRCPI FRCOG.**
Consultant Obstetrician and Gynaecologist
Royal Jubilee Maternity Service, Belfast., UK

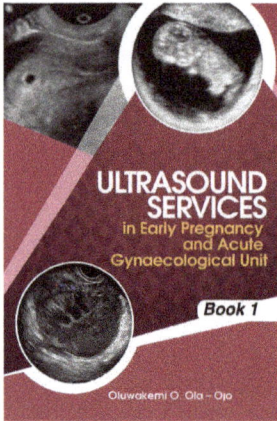

"*The scan pictures and details mentioned in the scan findings and techniques used make this book practical and easy to understand*".
"*Case reviews were interesting and logically approached*".
- Khaled Zaedi
Consultant Obstetrician and Gynecologist
EPAGU Consultant lead
Royal Free London NHS Trust

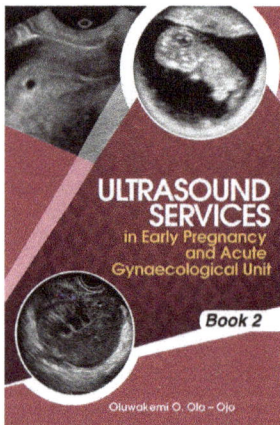

"*A comprehensive guide to gynecology /obstetrics ultrasound... a first reader for ultrasound trainees and references*"
- Phyllis Nsiah – Sarbeng
Then Radiology Registrar
Royal Free London NHS Trust

"*A very useful book both for those starting training and those seeking to update their knowledge base*".
- Peter Wylie
Consultant Radiologist
Royal Free London NHS Trust

"*A comprehensive guide to gynecology /obstetrics ultrasound... a first reader for ultrasound trainees and references*"
- Phyllis Nsiah – Sarbeng
Then Radiology Registrar
Royal Free London NHS Trust

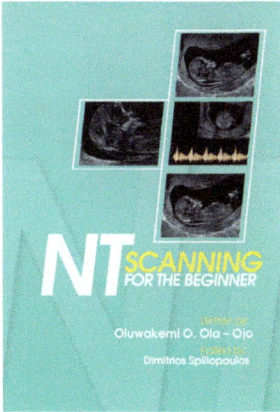

NT Scanning for the Beginner, is a book written by Oluwakemi Ola-Ojo, a trained and practising Radiographer/Ultrasonographer with years of experience.

The book simplifies NT scanning in the UK NHS using over 450 high quality resolution images in pictorial form and in addition, presents a number of cases with a brief explanation of each.

The opening chapter of the book gives an introduction on why it was written and what to expect from it. It itemizes the requirements for NT Scanning and the possible challenges the Ultrasonographer may face in the discharge of his/her duties. The contents of the book, which is captured in six chapters, covers other topics such as; quick anatomy check, types of tests including non invasive prenatal testing, documentation of the examinations, multiple pregnancies, nuchal cord, ductus venosus and the criteria of what makes good NT and CRL measurements, amongst others. Forty cases of abnormalities and variants are presented in the last chapter.

NT Scanning for the Beginner is a great handbook for the beginner in NT scanning and an excellent resource in ultrasound and obstetrics departments. Its simple layout makes it a good referral resource and ready manual in organised learning.

The book, which comes in a colorful and well-designed cover, will no doubt invite students and practitioners in the field to read. It is highly recommended!

Index

www.ingramcontent.com/pod-product-compliance
Lightning Source LLC
Chambersburg PA
CBHW050105220326
41598CB00043B/7393